Who Betrayed John Rittmeister?

Who Betrayed John Rittmeister? unravels the mystery of betrayal, resistance and psychoanalysis in the shadow of Nazi Berlin.

Rickels delves into the enigmatic circumstances surrounding the arrest and execution of John Rittmeister, a psychoanalyst and member of the resistance group *Rote Kapelle*. Through meticulous research and close readings of the works of Rittmeister's colleagues and his close friend Werner Krauss, Rickels uncovers the complex interplay of psychoanalysis, political resistance and survival under the Third Reich. The book explores the adaptation of psychoanalysis to the Nazi regime, the eclectic therapies of the Göring Institute, and the haunting legacy of betrayal. At its heart, the narrative examines Krauss's fictionalized account of their resistance efforts, offering a profound lens into the psychological and linguistic underpinnings of National Socialism.

This book is essential for readers interested in the history of psychoanalysis, the Third Reich and modern Germany. It will captivate graduate students, scholars in the humanities and those apprenticed to analytic theory, as well as art world enthusiasts drawn to Rickels' unique interdisciplinary approach.

Laurence A. Rickels analyses the condition of "unmourning" in literature, film, philosophy and psychoanalysis across his collected work of 15 publications, beginning with *Aberrations of Mourning* (1988). He dislodged this concept from the traditional opposition between successful mourning and melancholia. Psychoanalysis, the Frankfurt School and deconstruction inform his perspective.

History of Psychoanalysis

Series Editor
Peter L. Rudnytsky

This series seeks to present outstanding new books that illuminate any aspect of the history of psychoanalysis from its earliest days to the present, and to reintroduce classic texts to contemporary readers.

Other titles in the series:

Sigmund Freud's Inner Divisions
Personal and Theoretical
Ken Fuchsman

Sigmund Freud on the Way to Paris, 1873–1885
Foundations of Psychoanalysis
Giosuè Ghisalberti

Reading Freud's Beyond the Pleasure Principle
Trauma and Life
Herman Westerink

Between Genius and Tragedy
A Psychoanalytic Portrait of Viktor Tausk
Francisco Balbuena Rivera

The Psychoanalysis of Nazism
Language and the Unconscious in the Third Reich
Laurence A. Rickels

Who Betrayed John Rittmeister?
A Psychoanalytic Mystery from Nazi Berlin
Laurence A. Rickels

For further information about this series please visit https://www.routledge.com/The-History-of-Psychoanalysis-Series/book-series/KARNHIPSY

“Laurence Rickels has been a guiding beacon for me for two decades now. Nobody thinks the intersection of media and mourning better, or more lucidly argues for the place of trauma at the centre of our understanding of history and the arts.”

Tom McCarthy

“This book widens the understanding of the complex and contradictory motives of psychoanalysts and scientists remaining in Nazi Germany and being forced to cope with it.”

Ludger Hermanns, Psychoanalyst in private practice in Berlin and member of the Karl Abraham Institute

“On 13 May 1943, the neurologist and psychoanalyst John Rittmeister was beheaded by the Nazis in Plötzensee Prison in Berlin following charges of high treason and favouring the enemy. His resistance and fate made him something of an icon in the post-war reconstruction of psychoanalysis in Germany. His story was complex, historically, politically, and ethically. Left leaning, Rittmeiseter had been affiliated with both the notorious Göring Institute and the anti-fascist resistance group Rote Kapelle (Red Orchestra). In exploring Rittmeister’s fate, Laurence Rickels, the acclaimed historian of psychoanalysis in Nazi Germany, reopens this ‘cold case’, challenges previous reconstructions of the events, and offers new insights into his betrayal. In doing so, Rickels also reveals hitherto largely hidden sequelae of these events in a scandal in Brasil involving analytic training, torture, and the transmission of unacknowledged Nazi legacies. Building on close readings of archival research, clinical writings, postwar institutional histories, and literary fiction, Rickels has produced a nuanced work that is both a significant contribution to psychoanalytic history and at the same time a gripping detective/true crime page turner.”

Roger Willoughby, Oxford Brookes University, clinical psychologist and historian of psychoanalysis, Gradiva Award winner, author of Masud Khan: The Myth and the Reality *(2005) and* Freud’s British Family: Reclaiming Lost Lives in Manchester and London *(2024), and co-editor of historiesofpsychoanalysis.com*

Who Betrayed John Rittmeister?

A Psychoanalytic Mystery from Nazi Berlin

Laurence A. Rickels

Routledge
Taylor & Francis Group
LONDON AND NEW YORK

Designed cover image: *I Confess* (2011) by Margarete Hahner

First published 2027
by Routledge
4 Park Square, Milton Park, Abingdon, Oxon OX14 4RN

and by Routledge
605 Third Avenue, New York, NY 10158

Routledge is an imprint of the Taylor & Francis Group, an informa business

British Library Cataloguing-in-Publication Data
A catalogue record for this book is available from the British Library

ISBN: 9781041354345 (hbk)
ISBN: 9781041354338 (pbk)
ISBN: 9781003797708 (ebk)

DOI: 10.4324/9781003797708

Typeset in Times New Roman
by codeMantra

Contents

Acknowledgments

When you overstay your welcome at an institution, a university or a university press, it's as hard to move on as it is to reignite the honeymoon phase. I breached one impasse by accepting a professorship at the Academy of Fine Arts, Karlsruhe. "My" press, however, I realized only later, dropped me when I moved to Germany. While I learned to rely on the kindness of stranger presses, when I finally wrapped this genealogy of German-language psychoanalysis I felt its publication required a sturdier platform with an established psychoanalytic list.

My heartfelt thanks to Susannah Frearson for supporting this study. Although I wasn't sure that her interest would be enough, her diplomacy or resolve prevailed. After she arranged for two of the three books comprising my genealogy to go out for review, she went on maternity leave, a parallel that I tried seeing as good luck. Truth is that I was her other infant. While I did my best to hold back irrational feelings of dependency and abandonment, I must apologize to as much as acknowledge Eleanor Taylor, Saloni Singhania, and Tom Bedford, who were so helpful in the assembly and shaping of the constituent parts of this book.

Thank you, Tom McCarthy, for the generous endorsement. I'm grateful as well to another close friend, artist Margarete Hahner, for the use of her painting on the book's cover. My gratitude to my partner Alex Muñoz is as great as all that he had to pack away while I was trying 24/7 to catch up with my good fortune.

Introduction

This study was inaugurated by a scandal in Brazilian psychoanalysis or rather by my delayed cognizance of it. During the Brazilian dictatorship, the medical doctor Amilcar Lobo, an analytic candidate at the first institute in Rio de Janeiro to be recognized by the International Association of Psychoanalysis, was assisting in torture interrogations of political prisoners. A tradition of training, which does count as delegation in psychoanalysis, linked him through his didactic analyst, Leao Cabernite, to Werner Kemper, Cabernite's didactic analyst. After the war a site visit to Berlin by British analyst John Rickman had pronounced Kemper clear of complicity with the Nazi ideology. Ernest Jones agreed and decided to send him down to Rio to establish in his capacity as teaching and training analyst a bona fide psychoanalytic institute there. The scandal, which surfaced following Kemper's return to West Germany two decades later, came to be judged a delegation of what I dared name "Nazi psychoanalysis."

I would have liked to salute the judgment call as the confirmation of my own work, but the ease with which a deep commitment to National Socialism was uncovered in the work and life of Kemper made me ill at ease. Specifically, they charged him complicit in the betrayal, imprisonment and execution of John Rittmeister, his colleague and didactic analysand. Stepping to the side of history to pursue psychohistory would be understandable. But in journalistically or academically forthright pronouncements about the recent historical past, the international psychoanalysts who signed in could be as ignorant and careless as they were eager to see their faulty judgments in print. Time to remember that beyond the uncanny coupling I was after in the title of my 2002 book I was also following the lead of the psychotic patients on record who overheard in "Nazi" "not see." The sense or direction of "Nazi psychoanalysis" lies in "not seeing" the history of psychoanalysis, an impasse the analysts were acting out around the Brazilian scandal. Helena Besserman Vianna, who wrote the book on it, when called to account for inaccuracies in her presentation of the facts, answered that she hadn't intended to write a scholarly study.[1]

In the scandal's receiving area, largely shaped by Besserman Vianna's book, *The Politics of Psychoanalysis in the Face of Dictatorship and Torture: Don't Tell Anyone* (my translation of the title of the French translation), the commentary

DOI: 10.4324/9781003797708-1

ran that German analysts like Kemper were only fooling themselves when they claimed that by staying behind in the Third Reich, they were engaged in securing under the cover of adaptation the continued existence of psychoanalysis in and for Germany. Lobo's crime and Cabernite's cover-up were judged a wrap with a transgenerational transmission going back to the German Institute for Psychological Research and Psychotherapy, also known as the Göring Institute, a nickname owed to the man in charge, Matthias Göring, a psychiatrist and Adlerian therapist and the cousin of Hermann.

Saving psychoanalysis may well have been an illusion in Nazi Berlin, even a self-deception, one that helped the adjustment go down. But it's also more complicated and layered, reflecting, for example, the input of the former constituency as well. Michael Schröter argues that the idea of saving true psychoanalysis was championed by the Jewish émigrés who saw themselves persecuted as Jews *and* as psychoanalysts. At the Lucerne conference in 1934 the expected international objections to the *Gleichschaltung* (the forced conformity or synchronization) of the German Psychoanalytic Society (DPG) just didn't happen. When Max Eitingon quit the DPG to protest the discriminatory exclusion of the Jewish members, he arranged that the disbarred colleagues could still qualify for direct membership in the International Association. It followed that they viewed themselves as the carriers of true psychoanalysis.[2] Did the German psychoanalysts who stayed behind unwittingly render the Göring Institute in turn the hub of an uncanny continuity in the history of analytic psychotherapy as well as in the history of modernism? Or was the continuity already up and running in the Nazi readiness to hold on to psychoanalysis by any other name?[3]

For this study I am presenting works by the analytic colleagues of John Rittmeister in Nazi Berlin, those published between 1933 and 1945, as well as works that appeared postwar if composed during the Third Reich.[4] I commence with Kemper and acquit him of the indictment. But was he a good analyst? In the lineup of his books, he seems competent, but in the articles, like those published right after the war, which were based on presentations at the Göring Institute, he rises to the occasion a convincing analyst, and at times his presentation of a case is truly inspired. But that fits the bill for many analytic authors whose publications, unlike Kemper's efforts, are well-placed on the shelf of the history and study of their discipline.

That Otto Fenichel was Kemper's close colleague is more than forgotten.[5] Although Fenichel took offense that Kemper did not try to keep in touch (which is understandable given the exile's automatic inclusion of his correspondence in the circular he published, the *Rundbriefe*) he also made it clear that he valued his former colleague's work and talent. But by remaining behind, the German analysts like Kemper cut themselves off from the continuity and community of international psychoanalysis and remain today missing from its history.

In *Nazi Psychoanalysis*, I chose to read the extent of Freud's influence in the Third Reich outside the oeuvres of the psychoanalysts, thereby inadvertently joining in the devaluation of the work of the proper heirs of this influence, a corpus relegated a long time ago, certainly internationally, not to the archival vault but to the trash heap of history.

In adapting to the bad situation and to promote their field, the German psychoanalysts in Nazi Berlin became adept at finding loopholes in the loopy ideology. They found ways to get around the prohibitions and through the requirements. The analytic authors not only left out key terms or found synonyms but even inserted buzzwords from the new order. Although Kemper's colleague Käthe Dräger singled out his presentations at the Göring Institute, five of which were published as articles during the immediate postwar period, as proof that analytic work was still possible in the Third Reich, she also noted that in one of his books that appeared at that time the sleight of hand strategy or style was so heavy-handed that she was hard pressed to consider it still psychoanalytic.[6]

In the 1942 book Dräger refers to, Kemper underscores that a client selected for depth psychological treatment couldn't be the congenitally inferior type deserving of being sorted out.[7] We stand here before the largest construct of analytic compromise or camouflage at the Göring Institute. Felix Boehm, who governed what was left of psychoanalysis together with Carl Müller-Braunschweig after Max Eitingon stepped down, had a knack for recommending the application of analytic knowhow to the populations triggering official anxiety, notably war neurotics, criminals and homosexuals. Whenever analysts pitched in and offered expert counsel in the decision making about and the sorting out of the untreatables, the belief in the curability of "neurosis" was also being patched in. There were Nazi authorities who wanted to hear that anyone of good Aryan stock could be returned to Germany's forward march into the future.[8]

In the guidelines that the analysts at the Göring Institute helped formulate for military psychiatrists at the front, there was the proviso that soldiers sent back to Berlin for treatment, should they prove incurable, would be given back to the military for special handling.[9] Although she doesn't play a role in the study proper because she didn't publish, psychoanalyst Ingeborg Kath, who after 1933 was a secret communist, did, in a postwar interview, elaborate on her leading role in selecting defectives for euthanasia, which allowed her to save as many as possible, only letting go those patients "who were going to die anyway."[10]

In a 1944 letter Kemper advised his Viennese colleague August Aichhorn how the analysts in Berlin had to camouflage the entire "libido-theoretical system of coordinates." That's why over all these years one helped oneself out with a procedure that was "linguistically creative."[11] Circumlocutions that were used, Kemper writes, included *Trotzphase* (defiance phase) for the anal phase, *reife Form der Sexualität* (mature form of sexuality) for *Genitalprimat* (genital primacy), *Mundwelt* (mouth world) for the oral phase. Detours also had to be taken around the concepts of infantile sexuality, incest and the castration complex. And yet a cursory glance at the institute's journal shows that over the years it was possible to refer in print to all that Kemper cites as taboo. It's true that in 1944 the tolerance shown depth psychology was curtailed in the wake of Rittmeister's execution for treason the year before. Kemper replaced Rittmeister as the director of the clinic and it is from this vantage that he advises Aichhorn. However, from 1933 onward, it was also always the case that special care was taken in supervising the spoken language of exchange in which the psychoanalysts met with representatives of the other approaches.

Not able to detect among Kemper and his colleagues the culprit in this mystery, I began examining works by a non-analyst, Werner Krauss, looking to find an inscription therein of the fate of his close friend and fellow member of the resistance.[12] Like his GDR academic colleague Victor Klemperer, Krauss championed a philological and literary-critical approach to studying Nazi Germany. During his imprisonment in the Third Reich Krauss wrote under the cover of a scholarly study, which he was permitted to pursue in his cell, a novel, *PLN. Die Passionen der halykonischen Seele* (PLN. The Passions of the Halyconian Soul), in which he fictionalized his and Rittmeister's sojourn in the resistance.

In this literary parody, Krauss novelizes the Third Reich by taking apart and taking part in its faux languages. If there is hope in a language satire like *PLN*, then it must be placed, as Krauss explicitly does, in adolescence.[13] While he was preparing *PLN* for publication in the immediate postwar period, Krauss also wrote an essay on the condition of the German language that is to my mind the best analysis of the languages of the Third Reich, in which he attends to the surprising role of emo-teen idioms, which, through total-war mobilization, became the predominant slang of the soldiers.[14]

Herbert Marcuse touched down briefly on the terrain of Krauss's theorization in a review of two publications in Nazi Germany dedicated to the psychology of *Ganzheit*, a German word for totality. Marcuse highlights in the academic language being used, abused or recycled, specifically through many slight variations on the term *Ganzheit*, the condition of a language that must infuse an atmosphere of distinction where there can be none.

> Concerning the development of the basic concepts of totality psychology, one notes in the first place a manipulation of the words totality, whole, and structure, which lets the concepts turn circles faster and faster, without ever quitting the neutral gear (*Leerlauf*). With differentiations like "*Vollganzqualitäten*" ("fully total qualities"), "*Sonderganzqualitäten*" ("special total qualities"), "*Gesamtganzheit*" ("complete totality") etc., psychic phenomena and structures are to be described. The "*Gesamtbild*" ("complete picture") of the psyche, which these concepts grasp, looks, then, like this.[15]

Marcuse's posture of pointing out like the boy seeing through the emperor's new clothes what is manifestly absurd is akin to the sensibility of Berlin slang, in which the adverb *ganz*, completely, totally, was made to rhyme with the same-sounding noun *Gans*, meaning goose. The common affirmation, *Du hast ganz recht*, you are completely correct, can be slightly displaced as *Du Gans hast recht*, you goose are correct. It is this strand of cynicism that Krauss judged the vital supplement energizing the official stance and high discourse of Nazi Germany.

I hope that with this study I have done my share in rescuing the status of Werner Krauss's fictional and scholarly oeuvre from the accidental, incidental oblivion resulting from too many German histories. In the early days of the GDR, Krauss was no doubt obliged to publish his prison novel as the document of his own heroic resistance to National Socialism. But it remained overlooked and underrated on both sides of the German divide. Even though or especially because there is something uncompletable about it, *PLN* is to my mind the best documentation, from the inside out, from its language to its group psychology, of the National Socialist state (of mind). Of his several fiction attempts, only *PLN* was published in Krauss's lifetime. Still under the cover of his scholarly efforts, in the meantime as professor in the GDR, Krauss composed three more complete works of fiction.

The first was a sci-fi novel, *Die nabellose Welt* (The World Without a Navel), which he pursued in tandem with research on the related (but not identical) genre of fantastic voyages to utopia. His second try yielded a drama, *The Counterfeiter*, an intimate intrigue among couples in the style of Luis Buñuel or Edward Albee. The final trial was a diary novel, an offshoot of his scholarly interest in the work and life of Henri-Frédéric Amiel.

A cliché of raised eyebrows that characterizes the psychiatrist Eurylos in *PLN* (clearly Rittmeister's stand-in vis-à-vis the protagonist, Schnipfmeier, who represents Krauss) also enters into the physiognomy of the robots in Outer Space, which are associated with psychiatric care. At the close of *The Counterfeiter* it is a psychiatrist hailing from the recent past who commits the GDR author to an institution. In the final work, "Krauss" the diarist, is haunted by a ghostly voice amid his quasi-fictionalized entries. The voice-over belongs to Dr. W.R., and in the acronym of his moniker the names of the friends overlap or rather one incorporates the other. "Krauss" is delivered of the inner reality of their intertwining only upon the dog Knax's death. Krauss was an unmourner in the setting of pet grief (or he learned from his animals the litter of the law of survival): each dog he kept was always the same breed and always named Knax. In this final fictionalization of Krauss's life in diary entries, death happens to one Knax only and once and for all: the ghostly voice-over (which already beset Krauss's self-portrait in *PLN*) is over.

The idiom of urban youth marching as to war becomes the theme of adolescence in Krauss's subsequent fiction attempts. Conceived as being between the rock of psychopathy and the hard place of the schizoid state, youth is the evolutionary missing link that will not be ignored in the face of the revolutionary progress of socialism, extending all the way to Outer Space in *Die nabellose Welt*, and rebounding back to watch over the diary novel's entries about cute criminality. Krauss concludes that socialism dismisses at its own peril the rebellion of youth without a cause as residually prerevolutionary.

Intertwined with Krauss's work of mourning, which was tried and tried again, and then thrown to the dogs, we find, beginning in *PLN*, a tribute to *Don Quixote* and its own language combustion between an empty discourse elevated out of historical context and a more spontaneous idiom, folk wisdom running on empty, like the pun-slinging innovations lifted from the streets of Berlin and sent, via mobilization, to all the fronts of global warfare. One year into the Nazi dictatorship, Helene Deutsch intervened with a study of Don Quixote and Sancho Panza, nominating their duo dynamic, as does Krauss, as a more fitting vantage on the fascist state than Faustian daredevilry. If Don Quixote had been able to attract many Sancho Panzas to prop up his run on empty, she advises, he could have been a *Führer*. My book closes on a postmodern subgenre of Quixotic jousting with the aftershocks of the Nazi-psychoanalytic era in works by Kathy Acker and Robert Bolaño.

Notes

1 See Hans Füchner, "Psychoanalytiker, Mitläufer, Nazi, Gestapomann, militanter Marxist? Der Fall Werner Kemper," www.psychoanalyse.lu, November 2011, 52 pp. Besserman Vianna doggedly held onto the view that Kemper and Boehm were the analytic leaders at the Göring Institute who carried out the adjustment of Freud's science to fit the Nazi ideology. Let the record show that of the analysts who remained in Nazi Berlin after 1933, becoming members subsequently of the Göring Institute, one was a Nazi party member; two were communists, one actively engaged in maintaining undercover the organization of the non-Stalinist group; two were Marxists, one joining the Red Orchestra, the other saving up for his new beginning in the GDR.

2 Michael Schröter, "'Hier läuft alles zur Zufriedenheit, abgesehen von den Verlusten…' Die Deutsche Psychoanalytische Gesellschaft 1933–1936," *PSYCHE*, 63 (2009), 1085–1130; here: 1119–1120.

3 The policy of the Nazis was hardly uniform but buoyed up by rivalry among factions. Overall, however, a certain *Realpolitik* (the German word for "common sense" in a military setting) which sought to use whatever worked to fortify the fronts of the total war predominated. That psychoanalysis "worked" was on record with the military authorities owing to its good rep in treating war neurosis during World War One. Add to that the new emphasis on a psychologization of the conduct of war to make up for the amateur hour of their propagandists during World War One and we can see already in the 1920s evidence of an availability if not for psychoanalysis itself, then for the "reversal of psychoanalysis" that Adorno touted.

4 While I also consult on occasion work by the colleagues who emigrated, I do not give complete readings of their oeuvres. Regarding my main cast of characters, I allowed myself occasional exceptions. Ada Müller-Braunschweig published in 1930 an essay on problems faced in the upbringing of her son Hans. That it throws a high beam upon the analytically enlightened household a few years prior to the Nazi takeover fits the cultural anthropology trajectory of this study. And although the article counts as early by the parameters I set for myself, it was her last publication before devoting herself entirely to clinical practice. Little Hans, moreover, was destined to become a postwar analyst.

5 In his already cited article on "the case of Kemper," Füchner devotes a section to documenting the relationship between Fenichel and Kemper.

6 In the catalogue to the exhibition that accompanied the Hamburg conference of the International Psychoanalytical Association, *"Hier geht das Leben auf eine sehr merkwürdige Weise weiter…" Zur Psychoanalyse in Deutschland*, ed. Karen Brecht, Volker Friedrich, Ludger M. Hermmans, Isidor J. Kaminer, Dierk H. Juelich (Hamburg: Verlag

Michael Kellner, 1985), Kemper's camouflage language in his Third Reich publications is characterized as arguing at times in ways that implicitly agreed with Nazi ideas (150). "Kemper's own covertly analytic work in this period, *Disturbances in Women of the Capacity for Love*, was finally undecodable as analytic by his colleague Käthe Dräger: 'When you read Kemper's book you get the impression that in it psychoanalysis has fallen out through the grid'" (*Nazi Psychoanalysis*, volume one, 26).

7 *Die Störung der Liebesfähigkeit beim Weibe* (Leipzig: Thieme), 81–82. Representing the director Matthias Göring, Kemper helped compose the guidelines for military psychiatrists at the front on the important task of recognizing psychic reactions ASAP to forestall their epidemic spread, which had been the case with shell shock. Soldiers judged defective were assigned to a Strafkompanie (a punishment company) which was often sent on a suicide mission. But soldiers judged weakened in their resistance were first brought back from the front for psychotherapeutic treatment. If that failed, the assignment to a Stafkompanie was waiting. *"Hier geht das Leben auf eine sehr merkwürdige Weise weiter...,"* 152.

8 A *Diagnosenschema* (a diagnostic outline) had to be worked out at the Göring Institute to establish what counted as untreatable psychopathy. According to Andreas Peglau, *Unpolitische Wissenschaft? Wilhlem Reich und die Psychoanalyse im Nationalsozialismus* (Gießen: Psychosozial Verlag, 2013), 448–449, present and accounted for at this worktable were the non-identified psychologists, Schultz and Hattingberg, the ex-Jungian Rittmeister, the Jungians Kranefeldt and Achelis, the Adlerians Göring and Edgar Herzog, the revisionist Freudian Schultz-Hencke, and the Freudians Boehm, Kemper, and Müller-Braunschweig. The results were presented in 1940. Speaking for the group effort, Schultz gives the example of a diagnosis that's a death verdict: degenerate hysteria (*Entartungshysterie*), which is inherited and untreatable.

9 As we'll see, in his postwar interrogation by John Rickman, Felix Boehm boasts that he determined who among the malingerers could stay and who had to go. But there's a good chance that, impatient with the British invasion, Boehm was flashing Rickman with omnipotence. An Allied trajectory of the traumatic history of World War Two is another demo of utilitarianism. We do know that the Allies could not always intervene while reading along with the Germans their Enigma-encoded instructions. If they had, it was feared, the Nazis might have figured out that their code was cracked.

10 I first discovered the quote in her entry in the online archive *Psychoanalytikerinnen in Deutschland* and subsequently discovered the source, a conversation with Regine Lockot. See Lockot, *Die Reinigung der Psychoanalyse. Die Deutsche Psychoanalytische Gesellschaft im Spiegel von Dokumenten und Zeitzeugen (1933–1951)* (Tübingen: Edition Diskord, 1994), 78. "Going to Die Anyway" and "Almost Never" could be alternate titles for this genealogy.

11 Cited in Peglau, 472. I cite regularly from this study not only because it was the last in the long series of histories that I read and reread. It oddly demonstrates what an involvement with Reich can inspire in the capacity for history. Many authors have approached the Nazi era of psychoanalysis through Reich's exclusion from his field, his party, and so on. While his character armor is one of the conceptoids circulating in psychoanalysis today, not even through overvaluation can Reich be ratcheted up to a position that's key to understanding, promulgating, or even revising Freud's science.

12 Although not an analyst, Krauss was steeped in the culture of psychoanalysis and analytic therapy, even following Rittmeister into analysis with Hans von Hattingberg. Typical of German-language authors at the time he feared that analytic knowledge and self-knowledge would lead to a diminishment of his talent.

13 In 1991, during the run of the reconstructed Degenerate Art Exhibition at LACMA, high school students on a class trip often didn't advance beyond the Introductory Gallery

where clips from Riefenstahl movies were shown for the historical record. It takes one to know one, even when the other one hails from a condemned past. Adolescence or rather *Jugend* (youth) occupied the center stage of Nazi ideology, but to that end it was at once overvalorized and split off from itself.

14 "Notes on the Language of the Third Reich" (*MLN*, 137, 3 (April 2022), 586–600) was my advance preview of the import I uncover between the bookends of Krauss's *PLN* and his essay on the condition of the German language. However, "im Stich lassen," to abandon, was Krauss's example of how metaphor becomes a German phrase and not (this was a mistake in my article) a citation from the more recent footsoldier jargon during the Third Reich.

15 Herbert Marcuse, "Besprechung der psychologischen Bücher" (*Zeitschrift für Sozialforschung*, 5 (1936), 121–124. I read it among the appendices Wolfgang Bock includes in lieu of an afterword in *Dialektische Psychologie: Adornos Rezeption der Psychoanalyse* (Wiesbaden: Springer Verlag, 2018), 699–702; here: 700.

Part One

Who Betrayed JR?

Chapter 1

The Boys from Brazil

What came to be known in the literature as the "Lobo-Cabernite Affair" was up in lights as a special case of toxic spill from the adjustment disorder of German psychoanalysts adapting to the Nazi setting. It was in 1973 that the Argentine analyst Marie Langer received a clipping from a Brazilian underground resistance publication identifying a certain Brazilian doctor, Amilcar Lobo, as employed by the army on one of the torture teams that extracted information from political prisoners. Penciled in the margin, anonymously, was the further information that Dr. Lobo was an analytic candidate at the Psychoanalytic Society of Rio de Janeiro (also known as Rio One) and that he was the training analysand of the society's president, Dr. Leao Cabernite. Langer promptly made the identifications public in the newsletter *Cuestionamos*, which, although apparently easy enough to overlook, eventually did lead to controversy within the international psychoanalytic community in the second half of the 1990s.

Cabernite rejected the charge as libelous and received the backing of the International Psychoanalytical Association in the debacle he was facing down. Flashing back to the question recently raised by an associate of the Brazilian Psychoanalytic Society of Rio de Janeiro (also known as Rio Two) following a presentation by Wilfred Bion on the criteria for analytic candidacy, Cabernite submitted the registration form, on which those attending the Bion lecture had signed in, to a graphologist. For comparison check, Cabernite also gave the specialist a copy of the original handwritten notation he had obtained from Langer. The graphologist was able to identify Helena Besserman Vianna as the troublemaker.[1] In her 1994 book-length documentation of the affair, *Não conte a niguém... Contribuição à historia das sociedades psicanaliticas do Rio de Janeiro* (Don't Tell Anyone... Contribution to the History of the Psychoanalytic Societies of Rio de Janeiro), which had a major impact when it appeared in French translation in 1997,[2] although Besserman Vianna dismisses Cabernite's method of identification as symptomatically spurious, she has to admit that she was indeed the one who broke the story. Her safety had become less important than the common goal of saving psychoanalysis, which Cabernite energetically championed.[3]

Isolation and secrecy were the main themes of Wilfred Bion's Rio de Janeiro lectures delivered in 1974.[4] Before it's Besserman Vianna's turn to raise a question

DOI: 10.4324/9781003797708-3

during the discussion, someone else asks whether a patient who seeks treatment because he feels isolated can be taken seriously (168). In the back and forth that ensues another member of the audience intervenes with a lament and a double identification:

> The audience is in difficulties because you are trying to debate openly and frankly, and it finds itself in the position of the patient who says the only trouble with him is that he feels isolated. (169)

It's dangerous, Bion states, to assume "that psychoanalysts are people on whom you can put any job which no one else can do, and at which nobody else has succeeded" (175). The patient who feels isolated is a case in point: he doesn't know what to do and Bion can't do it for him: "If he is not prepared to use the knowledge he has, what is the good of my giving him any more?"

The next request for Bion's judgment and counsel, which was Besserman Vianna's, begs the question.

> A patient, referred to you by someone, comes to your consulting room; he says he wishes to have treatment – perhaps become an analyst – because he has difficulty in tolerating himself because he is a pervert, having committed atrocities against others. Would this case be within the minimum condition of acceptance?

Did the questioner expect Bion to slam the door in this hypothetical prospect's face? But Bion prefers to keep his audience guessing. The "minimum condition" is what the isolated audience is trying to get Bion to identify. But it's too much. I like to think that Bion was suspicious of the buzzword "pervert" and rallied from within his Freudian background to offer an acceptance of the hypothetical patient we can assume stands in for the torture perp. After analogizing the choosing of the client with the choice of bride or groom, Bion returns to the patient brought up in the last question. "I would say, 'If you wish, we can give analysis a trial!'" (176).

Why during Brazil's redemocratization during the 1980s was the case of Dr. Lobo, psychoanalyst, of all the many known cases of medical doctors participating in the torture of political prisoners, the most notorious? Hans Füchner answers the question by pointing to a dread of analytic abuse that can be found between the lines of the compact whereby the analysand submits to the rules, the scheduling and the frame.[5]

Lobo was publicly recognized and identified by several former political prisoners. He was party to the torture teamwork they had endured in what had come to be known as the House of Death. Before the 1980s were over, Lobo had given two tell-all interviews and published the memoirs of his double identity titled *The Hour of the Wolf, the Hour of the Sheep*.[6] While his name Lobo is also the word meaning "wolf," for his work in the House of Death he had used the pseudonym Carneiro, which means "sheep."[7]

Lobo simply did not recognize himself in the accusations of his alleged victims. Just like a physician he was always only standing by, ready to treat any damage done to a prisoner in a session of torture – in which he, the doctor, had not been directly involved. If the cured patient was hurt in the next session Lobo was still there to help and heal. He did admit, however, that one of his interventions could be interpreted by the uninformed as torture. Once between sessions he administered electroshocks to a political prisoner but did so only to reverse the symptom of paralysis in her legs.[8]

In response to Besserman Vianna's critical review of *The Hour of the Wolf, the Hour of the Sheep*,[9] in which she stressed the absence of shame in his account of his torture career, Lobo published a reply that took her to account for a naïve view of psychic reality:

> Dr. Helena Besserman Vianna writes that at no time have I shown shame at what I committed or witnessed in the four years I did military service. Nonetheless... she seems to forget that man has used torture and murder for thousands of years, ever since he organized into societies. Only a very short time ago, the Inquisition tortured and killed countless Jews and, a little over forty years ago, the German Nazi regime proceeded in the same manner. This is thus man in his total mental structure, and I am not ashamed to be one of them.[10]

Lobo summons prehistory (i.e., the recent past) in support of the institutional reversal of charges that Cabernite championed: Besserman Vianna rather than discuss a matter known to all at the institutes published an anonymous denunciation that called psychoanalysis into question.[11] The directors of the psychoanalytic societies in Rio de Janeiro moved against her once it was established by the handwriting analysis that she was the informant.[12]

In her review, Besserman Vianna judges Lobo's distortion of Freudian thinking symptomatic of those institutional tendencies in psychoanalysis that adapt Freud's science to "save psychoanalysis" in political settings where neutrality proves hard to maintain. But what about the propagandistic manner of Lobo's declarations styling between politics and psychosis? [13] Consider the way, for example, he homes in on Besserman Vianna's Jewishness and, transferentially, draws support for his counter charge from his secular identification with his Jewish fathers, both Freud and Cabernite.[14] His self-dramatization at the expense of the other's unconscious is reflected in the fantastic distortion of context in their exchange. Context is not only reduced, indeed displaced to the point of being lost, but also twisted one way, utterly cut off from any awareness of Lobo's own unconscious.

Besserman Vianna says he's an actor styling with a streak of psychosis that interlaces the loose ends of his personality (he himself repeatedly insists that he's not actually psychotic, which would be far worse). She observes that his discourse inheres in something basic to psychoanalysis, namely, the tension span between what's very extensive in its interpretations of the unconscious and what's very specific in the transference. The fantastic extensivity of interpretation addresses, in

Lobo's self-defense, thousands of years while the specifics of the transference can be date-marked forty years ago. Doesn't Lobo let in the ghost of the linguistic style of Nazi German, a spectral transmission across generations made manifest when in telling all in the second half of the 1980s he thinks he's preaching to the choir in and on prehistory?

It is in the setting of the Pax Americana, significantly, that Lobo goes beyond rationalization and borders on conspiracy theorizing and its syndications in psychosis. In *Hour of the Wolf, Hour of the Sheep*, he recalls a meeting early on in his military service with two men in civilian dress who spoke Brazilian Portuguese "with an accent that was fully American or English":

> They wanted to know about the possibility of my giving classes on techniques for interrogating political prisoners. They told me that the techniques used in Brazil were very primitive... They were proposing a new technique; an interrogation based purely in the psychological arena... They finished by justifying the search for a doctor who specialized in psychiatry, a professional who would have the largest possible background for preparing the Brazilian officials to adopt these new methods. (41–42)

Only a few pages have turned before Lobo questions his own sanity.

> I knew as a doctor and a psychoanalyst that I could well be the victim of some idea of persecution brought on by my experiences during the period of military service. The behavior of some of the officials in the Military Police and the DOI could easily drive one to formulate such ideas... On top of everything else, however, I wished to abandon these ominous activities and dedicate myself from then on to the work for and the study of others and myself.
>
> To what extent did my fantasies interfere with my awareness of the serious political reality that the country was passing through? The impossibility of establishing the limits between fantasy and reality drove me into feverish activity, physical and mental. (50)

That he came to identify with Christ is a trajectory of the same caliber as his rebuttal of Besserman Vianna in the name of mankind and mankind's unconscious politics.

Lobo's "martyrdom" commenced in 1982 with the first attempt on his life; the crucifixion happened in 1988 when the Regional Council of Medicine prohibited him from practicing medicine (111).

> I am not and never was religious. But the image of Christ flourishes in my thoughts. Christ was a man with ideas that questioned the structures of his time, and for this he was persecuted, imprisoned, tortured, and suffered martyrdom on the cross. On him fell the weight of the guilt feelings of a whole generation and he became the emblem of all those persecuted by institutionalized evil. (109–110)

The secular Passion isn't trending toward psychosis while the political reality of Cold War conspiracy leaves him doubting his sanity. He tags this reality possibly his delusion. It is a viable, historically motivated kernel of reality supporting the hypothesis of a transmission of a secret between separate eras or iterations of a politically compromised discipline.[15]

Lobo doesn't entertain "fantasies of physical mistreatment of anyone;" nor did he ever "feel any pleasure in someone else's suffering."

> There came a time while I was serving at the quarters that I started playing a role, putting myself in a cold, distant and unfeeling position whenever encountering people who were greatly suffering during the disgraceful period that devastated the country. But when I left the quarters, I went into a deep depression. I would lock myself in the treatment room and stay there for a while, without being able to digest the horrors I witnessed. Besides, it would be impossible to maintain a personality that for half the day was obligated to live with torture and for the rest attended to clients empathically in a psychiatric office. (110–111)

Division of the day and the psyche is the opening theme he evokes citing Ingmar Bergman's words on the hour of the wolf.

Lobo closes with Aesop's fable of the wolf drinking from a brook and espying a sheep doing the same. The wolf warns the sheep that when he attacks, the water the sheep drinks will be besmirched. The logical sheep replies along the lines of one of Zeno's paradoxes that what the wolf threatens just isn't possible given the distance keeping them apart: he will always be at another point along the brook. Protesting that it's not his fault, his father made him do it, the wolf devours the sheep. "Since 1981 Brazilian society sees me as a wolf in sheep's clothing. I anxiously hope that before the end of my days the wolf will devour this sheep once and for all." And so, the memoir ends on Lobo's signature mix of non-sequiturs.

In her review of Lobo's memoir, Besserman-Vianna scours a mediocre talent that only feigns boundary issues in the service of narcissism, the service that's as big as history:

> It is true that the author, at a certain point in his memoirs, affirms, in no original way, the "impossibility of establishing the limits between fantasy and reality..." ... He goes about weaving questionable *truths*, in which he always shows himself to be the victim of the cruelty or incomprehension of others, while he is being a caring and generous *soul*.

Besserman Vianna speaks of his "perversity:" while relating a relay of planned bombings that he refused to carry out (including a bomb intended for her), he succumbs, as she puts it, to his "singular preoccupation with his own personal injury."

> And so, the wolf intends to go on confusing everyone until he has presented himself as the victim of power, exploited by the higher ranks, inert at the

command of organizers of torture. Suddenly, he manages to make faithful *colonels* submit to the requests of a simple *soldier*, that they don't throw bombs into offices.[16]

Filling in the blanks shot in the dark of suspicion, various international analysts, all of them late arrivals to the Brazilian affair, managed to exchange one secrecy or distortion for another. Better that all the analysts at the Göring Institute should be Nazi henchmen than that they appear to be analysts in an eclectic therapeutic setting like people one might know. What we are up against here is a remarkable, indeed pathogenic, lack of historical formation, even or especially in the mode of psychohistorical application and revalorization. But if the commenting clinicians decline guilt by association on behalf of Jones as well as Serge Lebovici (who was IPA president during the onset of the cover-up of the Lobo-Cabernite Affair), they still rather blithely accept as decoded the secret history postulated by Besserman Vianna and René Major. Kemper's complicity in murder becomes the secret transmitted as torture.

In his March 2000 response to Besserman Vianna's open charges against the IPA from 1973 right through the present, Robert Wallerstein, at the time president of the IPA, does a double mistake. To defend himself against Besserman Vianna's charge that he had taken considerable care not to mention the prehistory of the Lobo-Cabernite Affair, namely the role of Werner Kemper, Wallerstein points out that Kemper was already dead for some time when Cabernite was analyzing and covering for Lobo, which reflects a remarkably timely understanding of transference and is anyway dead wrong since Kemper's finitude back in Germany was just coming due at the time of the first leaks of Cabernite and Lobo's secret. Kemper died in 1975.

Then Wallerstein overcompensates by referring to Kemper (in the past prior to his move to Brazil) as a Nazi, in fact a Nazi party member, and even the director of the Göring Institute. He gets this from a "careful reading" of Geoffrey Cocks's standard study of psychotherapy in the Third Reich. According to my research records, and in accord with Cocks's study, none of that is true. However, it is that much more mind-boggling that Wallerstein doesn't want to overreach for a connection among an outright Nazi, his Jewish training analysand Cabernite, and, next generation, Cabernite's training analysand, the part time torturer, part time candidate for membership in a society of psychoanalysts.

> I am offended at the implication that I did not mention the Cabernite-Kemper connection because of some implied desire to whitewash Cabernite, the disciple of the Nazi, who in turn would employ Gestapo tactics on the basis of that identification. For my part, I have not impugned Besserman's motivations, as she has mine. (1032)[17]

In his preface to the French translation of Besserman Vianna's book, René Major argued that in the Caberinite-Lobo Affair what the third generation fulfills in the mode of acting out, the middle generation that holds the place of latency withholds while transmitting the first generation's secret or encrypted history. In 2000 Besserman Vianna gave a parenthetical summary of the transgenerational history: "(Kemper, director of the Göring Institute, is training analyst to Cabernite, who is of Jewish origin and who in turn is training analyst to Lobo, who becomes a torturer)."[18] This transmission model, derived from Nicolas Abraham and Maria Torok's theory of cryptonymy, postulates shame's hidden relationship to the ego ideal, which cannot but pass it on. Because Major's interpretation addresses in Lobo and his silent partners from around the world of official psychoanalysis the symptomatic third generation, the motivation or momentum of this reading is found, by implication and transmission, in the prehistory, which in her book Besserman Vianna handles carefully, implicitly, and just the same (it's inevitable) tendentiously.[19]

I am entering the evidence of a legacy of Nazi psychoanalysis under the title borrowed from Ira Levin's demonic novel and F.J. Schaffner's spy-chiller film adaptation. The boys, the DNA doubles of Hitler, must be hatched in family settings of the antisocial tendency, which went into making the original boy into the *Führer*. After many trials there appears to be one boy who qualifies. But that hope, the last to go, is lost in the showdown between the mission to be carried out and the mystery to be solved. *Doppelt hält besser*, a phrase that expresses something like double-stitched is more secure, also admits that double is not enough. We'll never know whether the construction of the boy's deprivation and antisocial tendency could have developed the doubling destiny of Hitler's DNA inside him. What falls short of the conspiracy between biology and biography hypothesized in Levin's fiction rises again with the prospect of a transferential genealogy binding Lobo back through two didactic analyses to the Göring Institute. But the Nazi doubles or triplets also don't transmit to, through, or in the Lobo-Cabernite affair. At the limit, as noted, Lobo styles his atmospheric evocations and commandments in a manner remarkably reminiscent of the language of the Third Reich.

When in 1946 Brazilian psychiatrists put in the request to the International Psychoanalytic Association that certified didactic analysts be sent to Rio de Janeiro to establish there a bona fide psychoanalytic research and training institute, Ernest Jones, then IPA president, selected first Mark Burke in 1948 and then, six months later, Werner Kemper. Burke, Jewish, had left Poland some time prior to the Nazi invasion and concluded his analytic training in Britain. His main distinction was that he was Kleinian. However, it's unclear that he even qualified as a training analyst and his psychic lability was legend.[20] It's unclear why Jones sent him. Was it in the spirit of postwar integration that he chose them both together? Kemper was associated with the Berlin psychoanalytic society since 1928. He was also one of the official analysts who after 1933 accepted compromise and adaptation in the alleged effort to save the original psychoanalytic institute with its world-famous clinic, which upon incorporation within the so-called Göring Institute in 1936 was still recognizably intact, becoming one of the cornerstones of the new institute.

No comment by the parties to the tension that in no time arose between Burke and Kemper and their students. Besserman Vianna notes that vague rumors surrounding their incompatibility were the only static coming down the receiving line of Kemper's historically unique dossier. In no time there were two IPA-approved psychoanalytic societies in Rio. Besserman Vianna's own psychoanalytic society, the one, I mean Rio Two, associated with Burke, closed ranks with Rio One in the foreground of the IPA's backing of Cabernite's counter charge against her of calumny. In 1975 her request for full society membership was turned down. She was furthermore informed that the society's decision was secret, registered only in a confidential file. She nevertheless pressed for a meeting with the society's governing council. At the secret meeting she saw the writing on her file lying on the table between them: she was charged, so far only internally, with denunciation of a torturer, a charge that if forwarded to the authorities could have sent her, too, to the House of Death.

Several months later Besserman Vianna declared that she was taking the Cabernite-Lobo case, as well as her own, to the IPA meeting in London, despite the repeated threats to her and her family. Upon her return the society swiftly proposed the swap of full membership for her promise to destroy the correspondence. She shook on it but kept the correspondence as proof and bartering chip for her own security.

Notes

1 The scandal aborted plans to hold the annual meeting of the International Association of Psychoanalysis in Rio de Janeiro, which would have made Cabernite the first South American president of the Association. That's another notch in the Werner Kemper legacy that was lost in the controversy.

2 Helena Besserman Vianna, *Politique de la psychanalyse face à la dictature et à la torture: N'en parlez à personne* (Paris: L'Harmattan, 1997). There were subsequent editions in 1998 and 2000.

3 That the consultation with a graphologist occasioned the strongest reaction is overdetermined. Graphology, as we'll see, is related to a secret of corruption and compromise in Kemper's career, one that doesn't, however, decode as his being or having been a National Socialist.

4 Wilfred Bion, *Brazilian Lectures: 1973, Sao Paolo; 1974, Rio de Janeiro* (London and New York: Routledge, 1990). Page references are given in the text.

5 Hans Füchner, "Politische Folter, Psychoanalyse und gesellschaftliche Macht. Anmerkungen zu einem brasilianischen Beispiel," *IWK-Mitteilungen*, 1 (1992), *Seelenmord – Psychosziale Aspekte der Folter*, 18–24.

6 Amilcar Lobo, *A Hora do lobo, a hora do careiro* (Petrópolis: Editora Vozes, 1989). Page references are given in the text. In working with this text written in a language I don't command, I hired way-back-when a UCLA graduate student to help. I'm sorry, but I no longer remember her name, nor could I find a trace in my checkbook etc. It was long ago. Karlheinz Barck kindly double checked the translations when I was at the center for the study of literature in Berlin where he was employed as Wissenschaftlicher Mitarbeiter. He also helped me with newspaper publications, notably Zenir Ventura's interview with Lobo, which appeared in *Jornal do Brasil* on September 14, 1986. I also relied on already translated quotations from the Portuguese sources that had already appeared in English-language articles. I owe Barck more than assistance with Portuguese texts.

He had been Werner Krauss's doctoral student in the GDR and helped me immeasurably in becoming a close reader of his mentor's work.

7 As Lobo underscores, Ingmar Bergman used the "hour of the wolf" as his special locution for a time of madness. It was the title for his sole horror movie, the 1968 *Hour of the Wolf*, which he wrote and directed. A debilitating awareness of going mad gives way to the stabilizing paranoid conviction that they are under the remote control of a cult on the other side of the island.

8 Lobo unwittingly touched here on the outer limit of traumatic neurosis in the setting of war which led to a widening of the scope of psychoanalysis as theory and therapy. It was a primal scene in the genealogy I wrapped in *Nazi Psychoanalysis*. By interpreting the limited efficacy of the faradic current treatments of shell-shocked soldiers, psychoanalysis advanced an inside view of a conflict that the torture or rather the uneven results of its treatment confirmed. What hurts more (and longer), the administered shock or being shot at? When Freud opened his second system and introduced the superego, he was doing the aftermath of his insight into the struggle between the peace ego and the war ego, which, as Freud foresaw in 1919, would advance psychoanalytic understanding and treatment across the borderline into psychosis. The good rep and rap bestowed on Freud's science as the treatment of choice for war neurosis was arguably the main reason the Nazi authorities realized they couldn't leave home to wage war without it.

9 Helena Besserman Vianna, "The Hour of Democracy; the psychoanalyst who denounced Amilcar Lobo's involvement in torture writes about his memoirs," *Jornal do Brasil* (September 30, 1989).

10 Lobo's response is included in the supplement "The Tortured Speak," *Jornal do Brasil* (September 14, 1986).

11 Lobo maintained that his didactic analyst as well as any number of other analysts at Rio One knew about his situation. He had repeatedly turned to his colleagues and teachers for guidance. Cabernite finally did offer to help his training analysand by finding a position for him in the United States. Lobo analyzes his inability to accept this offer in terms of the difficulties he experienced in childhood under the care of a stepmother for whose nurture he just wasn't available. See the interview, "The Psychoanalysis of Torture," published in *Jornal do Brasil* on September 14, 1986. In his confessional writing he sees himself as the victim. By naming names not only of victims but also of torturer colleagues in interviews and in his book, he found himself the target of two assassination attempts, one of which severely compromised his health.

12 See L. Cabernite's statement in "The Tortured Speak," appended to the interview "The Psychoanalysis of Torture."

13 Representing the Chicago group in 2000 at the Estates General of Psychoanalysis meeting in Paris, Besserman Vianna introduced her précis or update of the Cabernite-Lobo Affair via a theoretical frame she borrowed from the local talent on the shore of Lake Michigan, a professor moreover of German Studies. "Individual and collective predicaments and conflicts arise," according to her cover or paraphrase, "when there are changes in the fundamental matrix of the individuals' relations with social and institutional authority, and in the way each one responds to the demands of power and the so-called 'official' authorities." Those invested with power are invested up front with a symbolic mandate that, the paraphrase continues, "impregnates their identity in the community. In these cases, both the stability of the institution and the emotional balance of each of its members become subject to the social symbol attributed to them by way of names, titles, positions, honors and similar attributes." Besserman Vianna counsels, therefore, that for the history and future of psychoanalysis "transparent and always well-documented clarification of certain historical happenings" alone can lead to an essential understanding of the responsibilities involved in arbitrary or despotic acts of political consequence. Otherwise, ethical predicaments become via repetition

"trans-generational, due to the particularities inherent in transference and transmission in psychoanalysis." See Helena Besserman Vianna, "Ethical Predicaments in Psychoanalytical Institutions," which I consulted for my 2008 article on the Lobo-Cabernite Affair. At the time I found her lecture here: www.spdecaracas.com.ve/download/edt_197.txt. Like the psychotic and his delusional system, psychoanalysis too is largely on its own in a larger stateside setting, with as little backing by-and-large as individual artists who, according to Klaus Theweleit in *Buch der Könige* (Book of Kings), must operate as states within states to assert diplomatic immunities and other protections for their lines of production. The generation of societies and institutes – via the differences generated around the Lobo-Cabernite Affair there were by the end of the twentieth century no longer two (or three or four) but 20 psychoanalytic societies in Rio de Janeiro – could be seen as the measure of the lack of outer protection of psychoanalytic interests.

14 Lobo's interim wife Francys and her daughter Renata were Jewish, which was a problem when his inner emigration took them to the countryside (no Jewish schools out there). They separated (87). He insists that he's not anti-Semitic since he participated in the Jewish culture of psychoanalysis. But no more: the Jewish-influenced rules governing the Psychoanalytic Society were partly why he left. Its governance should be more democratic (92).

15 What the three involved in the kinship system of the transference that allegedly brought home a Nazi secret all had in common, as postwar as the episode with American-accented officials, was an interest in analytic group therapy. Kemper would have been familiar with and wary of the Adlerian community therapy and theory that was current at the Göring Institute. But like his colleagues in South America, he rallied to a genuinely psychoanalytic group therapy. Cabernite's research portfolio was minimal, but the main asset was his work in group psychotherapy. And Lobo reports that his early entry upon analytic psychotherapy was via a group therapy course he attended before he began training in psychoanalysis at the institute. The instructor, Ernesto La Porta, soon had Lobo, who was best in class, treating and supervising members of his team. Lucia Villela, "The Chalice of Silence and the Case that Refuses to Go Away," *Psychoanalytic Review*, 92, 6 (December 2005), 807–828; here: 827 n. 6.

16 In his memoir Lobo rejects one of Dr. Helena's statements to the press. Allegedly he followed her and, grabbing her attention, threatened her life should she continue with her denunciation. Lobo denies even knowing her personally and says that he would never act in such a way (78).

17 Hans Füchner opens his essay on the case of Kemper with Inaura Carneiro Leão's mortified recollection of Wallerstein's ahistorical and inept characterization of Kemper as a Nazi. A long list of these libelous references to Kemper's secret past could be compiled. Someone who should know better, Stephen Frosch, in "Psychoanalysis in Troubled Times: Conformism or Resistance?" invokes the study by James E. Goggin and Eileen Brockman Goggin to identify Kemper as a "collaborator with the Nazi Regime" (147). I can let that stand if the collaboration charge applies to all able bodied Germans who weren't engaging in political resistance, but it's not terribly differentiating nor is it historical. I also don't recall that the Goggins make this explicit claim. They do conclude that Kemper was another Zelig, though presumably not a Jewish impostor (205). The Frosch article is in *Psychology and Politics. Intersections of Science and Ideology in the History of Psy-Sciences*, ed. Anna Borgos, Frenc Erös, and Julia Gyimesi (Budapest and New York: CEU Press, 2019), 137–151.

18 "The Lobo-Cabernite Affair," *Journal of the American Psychoanalytic Association*, Letters, 48, 3 (2000), 1023–1029; here: 1026. The recurrence or its triggering might be found (or lost) in the memory or fantasy of Lobo's recruitment by US experts to use his psychological savvy to improve the efficacy of torture. In the interrogation sessions he

says that he never administered torture but only treated its side effects like analysts did decades before when sending soldiers back to the front.

19 In the first paragraph of their review of Besserman Vianna's book in French translation, Janine Piaget and Miguel A. Stamati write: "Cabernite's own analyst had been Werner Kemper, a psychoanalyst of Nazi ideology…," *Journal of the American Psychoanalytic Association*, 47, 3 (June 1, 1999), 961–964. I thought a more balanced reception was evident when Lucia Villela referred to Kemper as "one of the directors of the Göring Institute." But later Villela refers to Kemper two more times, first as "a former director of the Göring Institute," which still resonates with more than one director, then as "the director of the Göring Institute" ("The Chalice of Silence and the Case that Refuses to Go Away," 809, 820). Beginning in 1943, Kemper was the director of the institute's clinic.

20 Hans Füchner, "Mark Burke (1900–1975). Ein fast unbekannter Pionier der Psychoanalyse in Brasilien," *Luzifer-Amor. Zeitschrift zur Gescihte der Psychoanalyse*, 31, 62 (2018), 155–169.

Chapter 2

A Peculiar Form of Resistance

At the outset of a lifelong career of documenting the complicity of psychoanalysts with the dark side, Besserman Vianna wrote a clinical research paper, a requirement for institute membership, in which she contemplated a case from the paradoxical bounty of analytic work in Brazil under the dictatorship. Her 1974 article, "A Peculiar Form of Resistance to Psychoanalytical Treatment,"[1] which she first presented the year before at the 28th International Psychoanalytical Congress in Paris, was published in *The International Journal of Psychoanalysis* together with a discussion by Willy Baranger. It was a show of respect that Baranger, who famously formed an analytic power couple with his wife Madeleine Baranger, was selected to respond to her paper.[2]

Her patient, a wealthy industrialist, is Lobo's contemporary and his colleague in narcissistic disturbance, but her relationship to the former is staggered through resistance and transference, the specific work of analysis. In the first session, analyst and analysand explore his wish to be in control of all her scheduling, all her time, and interpret his difficulties in accepting any dependence, especially dependence on the analyst (441 col. 2). Session over and the patient starts acting out an alternate scheduling as though he cannot bide the time of the sessions, and the analytic frame could not but collide with the patient's aggrandized sense of his greater timeshare. Sessions are missed (he never contacts her about a change of plans) or diminished by late arrival. His insomnia gives him license to disrupt all schedules while finding time for deep sleep. In the epigraph to her paper Besserman Vianna cites Heraclitus on the difference between the waking state, a single, common world in which the subject adapts and follows a schedule, and sleep, which returns the subject to a world of his own.

Insomnia suggests deficiency or lack of sleep. But in her patient's case it's rather that he can't moderate his tendency to sleep without end, except by pulling an all-nighter. After a workday, he finds that he can fall asleep only if completely exhausted. So, he reads and plays patience. Passing out at the crack of dawn, he then sleeps soundly and continuously for at least 24 hours, but even for as long as 36 to 48 hours. If he wakes up in the daytime, he appears for the analytic session and then goes to work. If he's not up until the late afternoon, he stays up all night

DOI: 10.4324/9781003797708-4

to keep the appointment with his analyst. But because when it's time to sleep the patient can't sleep, and when he's supposed to be awake, he sleeps, his analytic appointment schedule becomes more miss than hit.

Although she doesn't clarify whether the onset of the sleep disturbance coincided with the analysis, the analytic frame in any event would have made this disturbance manifest (it was not his presenting problem). Besserman Vianna is justified in interpreting the pattern as a form of resistance. Not unusual for the 1970s the analysis was conducted at the border to psychosis. There is an affinity in the degree of narcissism between Besserman Vianna's two borderlines, the resistant patient and Lobo. But for the latter case of narcissism, which becomes manifest through Lobo's confessional discourse in the late 1980s, she has no transference time. How is Lobo's styling with psychosis to hide out on the dark side of human nature not borderline behavior? But if for her and Major what prompts Lobo's acting out isn't resonant with his own psychic reality, why, then, is the language itself not the message, the secret passage?

Baranger's only criticism of her case study is that her own input should have been underscored. "Envy and narcissism, we agree, but at the same time a specific system of exchanges in which the analyst also plays a role" (447 col. 1). What he circumscribes as her countertransference in the case study is her being triggered by lamenting self-recrimination, a response that has no place to go in her altercation with Lobo but which she contains within the relationship to her patient. When her sleep-in no-show patient complained in session "of his inability to succeed in life, calling himself weak and inferior and saying that he felt very disgusted with himself" (442 col. 1), Besserman Vianna brings the patient "face to face with the falseness of his lamentations, facing him with the actual relationship which he attacked, debased and made insufficient by his absences, although he attempted to explain them by the alteration in his sleep rhythm" (442 col. 1–2).

Commenting on her review of the literature, from Freud and Abraham to Klein and Rosenfeld, Baranger addresses the "evolution" of psychoanalysis in a force field of mutually determining changes in technique, theory and client population. Besserman Vianna's understanding of the patient's negative therapeutic reaction manifests "a theoretical detour, a going to-and-fro between theory and clinic," which is basic to the developmental history of psychoanalysis itself (446). Passing through the "theoretical detour," the alternation between theory and therapy, original concepts are not so much updated as diluted, by which he means that they gain in extension at the expense of their specificity (445 col. 2). This applies not only to the negative therapeutic reaction but to other analytic concepts as well (like acting out).

> We cannot help noting that the cut-through permitted by theory at the clinical level no longer encompasses Freud's former classification. After all, the negative therapeutic reaction is defined as a technical difficulty produced by envy and narcissism and capable of assuming the most varied forms. (446)

Besserman Vianna indeed relies in the analysis on Melanie Klein's concept of envy, which transfers the death drive from metapsychology to the in-session relationship.

> Envy made itself evident as a desire to destroy the object capable of giving something good to the patient by denying that he has any necessity of love, dependence, or interest for external objects. This denial the patient obtained by his altered rhythm of sleep. (442 col. 1)

The patient's insomnia is the excuse for a sleep irregularity that promotes extension of sleep time, his time share in the fantasy of union with the idealized breast (442 col. 1). His sleep pattern, which demands that all scheduling be wrapped around it, conceals both feelings of inferiority and sensations of triumph, ultimately over the analysis. He was "so powerful that no one, not even death – identified with-sleep – could help him, much less modify him" (442 col. 2).

Besserman Vianna sought to "show" the patient through their relationship

> that the stagnation of his activities through prolonged sleep served not only as a form of concealed triumph over the analyst and analysis, but also as a pretext for complaining about my incompetence to take care of him, and his own incompetence in facing life. (442 col. 2)

But the other side of her competence and his dependence was his omnipotence. Succumbing repeatedly to the "fantasy of giving life to himself, of being capable of taking care of himself without needing the help of anyone," the patient reacted to perceptions of the reality of his dependence on the analyst

> as if he would rather not exist, as if he would deny the fact of his own birth, taking refuge in sleep, in a way identified with death, but which essentially served to destroy any possibility of analytical success, as well as any success of his own in his work, in his creative capacity, or directly, in life. (443 col. 1)

Besserman Vianna interprets and seeks to contain as negative therapeutic reactions motivated by envy even "the patient's omnipotent attitudes that always resulted in the loss of his sense of reality and, without doubt, in the loss of his capacity to think and even exist" (443 col. 1). He's not psychotic – he's just her bother until he wakes up and realizes he wants the analysis to fail under his control.

Baranger points out that according to Freud's original concept the negative therapeutic reaction comes about "when the analyst feels sure that he understands the analysand, and when the latter shares this assurance." What looked like progress proves a setback: "through it the analysand frustrates the analyst's success and triumphs over him. It is a last resource on the part of the analysand: after all, he is still capable of making the analyst fail, even at the cost of his own failure" (446 col. 1). The resistance is the transference in such a case, which qualifies Besserman Vianna's reading of it as the hot mess of envy. Baranger underscores that what justifies Besserman Vianna's reading is the "masked feeling of triumph" she observes in her patient (446 col. 1).

Besserman Vianna concludes that after two years she was able to deliver the transferential relationship from the impasse of the insomnia defense.

> Each form of behaviour, each fact, could be – as we know it is – repeated, recalled, transformed, decomposed and recomposed, during treatment; new forms are always emerging, which, when put into new fields of utilization, offer new perspectives in the transferential process and in the attainment of insight. (443 col. 2)

Toward this end she was able to "strengthen the patient's ego, and in consequence, enable him to establish a better relationship with the analyst and with his own objects. I do not mean that the feeling of envy disappears, but that it probably acquires new contexts and formulations" (443 col. 2).

Bion set the stage for his Rio de Janeiro lectures by distinguishing between "just like" and "becoming" in the evaluation of analytic candidates. A candidate deemed poor by Bion could well be "like" a psychoanalyst: but that's not the same as becoming an analyst (78). Only the adolescent can, by accident, become a grown-up by busily trying to be just like a grown-up.

In lecture number two Bion addresses the thing itself that presses to be seen, felt or intuited in psychoanalysis. That thing involves the relationship, not the things related.

> It seems to me that this is something like… what Freud meant when he used the word "transference"; he was not just inventing a word; he was convinced that there was a thing itself which required naming in order to talk about it. (86)

The thing that required naming is neither the analyst's memory nor his desire, "the one being the future tense of the other" (88).[3] What it is is what the psychoanalyst has risked in formulating the new designation. In the act of new naming, he is in danger of evoking the "sensuous history" of the words he selects, rearranges or denies, which means that "as with a 'dead' metaphor carelessly used, its ghost begins to walk" (87). While in augmenting its vocabulary psychoanalysis borrows from other disciplines, in the session (in the transference) we must as much as possible "manufacture our means of communication while we are communicating" (89). Bion therefore identifies the session as inherently a chance for recovery from what courses through it: like the languages of adaptation to bad situations.

Notes

1 Helena Besserman Vianna, "A Peculiar Form of Resistance to Psychoanalytical Treatment," *The International Journal of Psychoanalysis*, 55 (1974), 439–444. Page references are given in the text.

2 Willy Baranger, "A Discussion of the Paper by Helena Besserman Vianna on 'A Peculiar Form of Resistance to Psychoanalytical Treatment,'" *The International Journal of Psychoanalysis*, 55 (1974), 445–447. Page references are given in the text.

The Barangers promoted the concept of the "bastion" in the analytic setting/session, the unconscious refuge of powerful fantasies of omnipotence that the patient will defend as resolutely as the melancholic his crypt.

3 "To remember, to foresee, to understand," Bion clarifies on pages 88–89, "may all be relevant and desirable, as for example when reading a book or participating in a lecture, but during the practice of psychoanalysis none of them is a valuable activity; they are breaches in the analytic frame of mind."

Chapter 3

Besserman Vianna and Rittmeister[1]

The committee at Rio Two that rejected Besserman Vianna's first application for full membership, when pressed by her for explanation, included the charge that she had plagiarized her 1974 article. The specificity of the committee's charge – not unoriginality but plagiarism – coming seemingly from nowhere, but symptomatizing incomplete mourning and improper burial, parallels in its severity the charge that she denounced a torturer. It is a wrap, I would argue, with the nimbus of haunting around Besserman Vianna's enactment of John Rittmeister's role in his missing place.

Rittmeister was Mr. Oblivious, moving to the capital of Nazi Germany to pursue a career in psychoanalysis while getting involved in a resistance group (no problem!). One cannot but wonder why Besserman Vianna remained in Rio as analyst at once politically committed to resistance to the dictatorship (and to its internalization within her profession) and equally committed to obtaining membership in a society willing to risk her life in exchange for good relations with the authorities. At this enigmatic point of impasse her political position of asking for it can be likened to that of John Rittmeister, who comes up in Besserman Vianna's and Major's accounts only in passing as ghostly accuser at the banquet of Kemper's unstoppable opportunism.

The young Hamburg-born psychiatrist left Switzerland for Berlin in 1937 not only because he had to go (the local authorities judged his left wing politics to be trouble) but also because he planned to train as a psychoanalyst at what he was not alone in still viewing as the leading institute for this purpose.[2] Amazingly, the first reason for the move was not registered by the Nazi German authorities, or perhaps they saw it cleared by the second resolution. In 1936 the German psychotherapies that had journeyed far away from Freud's science were prompted to return to their provenance and *Heimat*. They brought back the treasure of "Greater Psychoanalysis." Felix Boehm, the psychoanalyst who claimed to have negotiated the reunification in exchange for access to the facilities of the former analytic institute, saw in the reunion both a measure of protection for psychoanalysis and an opportunity for his discipline to reassert influence on the eclecticism that was, after all, part of its own history.

Because both Boehm and his closest colleague Carl Müller-Braunschweig were identified going into the merger as Freudian (and more importantly as the last of

DOI: 10.4324/9781003797708-5

the generation with personal ties to the founding father), Matthias Göring was wary of giving either one too much influence. His suspicion of psychoanalysis, which would be tempered by an appreciation of the clinical prowess of the analysts working at the institute's clinic,[3] reflects more his identification with Freud's outlaws (Adler and Jung) against the master's "orthodoxy" than a political stance like the racialist judgments of Nazi ideology. Just the same, while several Adlerians and many more Jungians were Nazis, only one analyst (whose connection with the institute was from a distance) joined the party.

What the Göring Institute was looking for was a colleague who commanded the therapeutic skills attributed to psychoanalysis, but who was committed less to Freud and more to "Greater Psychoanalysis." Enter Rittmeister, whose presentation at the Berlin Institute in 1937, "Die psychotherapeutische Aufgabe und der neue Humanismus" (The Task of Psychotherapy and the New Humanism), aligned the striving for an eclectic but unified German therapy with his own agenda.[4] Rittmeister gained the approval of the Institute where he was subsequently appointed director of the clinic.

In the strategically addressed text, which he composed already in 1935, Rittmeister argues for rigorous eclecticism in treating an obstacle course of polarities, supporting a relay of "bridges" between the developing ego and the environment (935), which he checks off quickly. He includes the "relationship to the other sex" (936), a remarkable reformulation in mature terms of the analytic prospect of sexual difference in childhood. He rests the litany on the equally remarkable bottom line of a "relationship between the ego and all others, between ego and death" (936). The check-off list introjects a stance that speaks to the Nazi ideology, but Rittmeister's discourse is overall way too sophisticated to be corralled inside such an adjustment.

The psychotherapist cannot provide a system for the patient whose autonomy is at stake. The schools of psychotherapy actively distinguishing themselves against each other attest to the difficulties in the basic setting common to them all, in which what is maintained and administered is, in Rittmeister's words, the very system of systemlessness or, rather, the acknowledgment of the unsystematicity of systems (936). The blocked relations that crowd out and shut down the patient's world must be revalorized as tasks. Via the overcoming of resistance and the raising of repressed materials to consciousness the obstructed tasks can be restored or inaugurated.

To illustrate the "anthropological strokes of the pendulum" in the psychotherapeutic process, Rittmeister turns to the Freudian and Jungian perspectives, commenting first on their divergent views of the provenance of symbols (937). For Freud they are created anew, beginning in early childhood, and continuing through the individual's instinctual clashes with the environment, that is, in the first place, with the family. For Jung they are "pre-existing ideas" hailing from the collective unconscious (937). Freud says complexes; Jung says archetypes.

His postulation of omnipresent quintessential archetypes notwithstanding, Jung carefully avoids the appearance of religion by viewing the collective unconscious as "the cellar beneath the cellar" or the "phylogenetic inheritance" (938). The prospect of a pragmatic-historical understanding of these secret powers and images is also not ruled out. And yet their postulation of a far more profound unconscious allows the Jungians to dismiss the mere unconscious of the Freudians, which Rittmeister likens to the children's playroom that, because they can't get past it, they turn into their lab space.

> While the combat zone of Jungian theory and analysis is crowded with spirits, angels, and demons and many other spectral beings, but also heroes, sorcerers, noble beings of every sort, the situation with Freud is more objective. The forces in question may be the same, but when they appear they are contained in test tubes, delivered of their dangerous poison and labelled. (938)

That modern psychotherapy is inherently an eclectic process is part of "the anthropological problem" (937). Not only do the patients experience themselves alternating between being object and being subject, at once unique and determined, but even the clinician is equally immersed in this unsettling setting (936). The anthropological perspective is only valuable, however, on the condition that it not get stuck on some sense known in advance and ascribed to "the" human, "but rather consider the biological-historical vantage point with its concrete particularities. Only then can an uncommitted anthropology of the individual human become a *humanism of decision* that sets itself concrete goals for the community" (936).

In his 1968 eulogy of Rittmeister, Werner Kemper, who was his didactic analyst and colleague in Nazi Berlin, singles out this article, which could not have been better designed as a pitch for acceptance at the eclectic Göring Institute, as the work that most fully discloses Rittmeister's character and attitude (*Einstellung*).[5] Kemper emphasizes the import of humanism in the place of the new: while analytic psychotherapy must for the time being remain an individual concern, beyond that there is the "humanist task" to apply the knowledge amassed in the course of countless individual cases to the practical alleviation of social distress and the suffering of the unprotected. Assessing the balancing act within the triad, Kemper gives Rittmeister credit for siding with the psychoanalysts: "Instead of finding a following and connection (*Anschluß*) among the well tolerated Jungians or the community psychologists, he decided to ally himself with our ostracized (*verfemte*) band of Freudians" (148 col. 2–149 col. 1).

Kemper is on the same page, in 1968, with *PSYCHE*'s revisionist history of psychoanalysis as one of the victims of the Third Reich. He offers the self-defense that the German analysts working at the Nazi Berlin institute were able by the authority of their associations with other clinics, hospitals and institutions to intervene indirectly but strategically and save many lives (149 col. 1). In outlining the paradox of this authority, he goes through the series of displacements and renamings that the analytic group underwent but pulled out of it each time still holding the key position of running the institute's clinic (149 col. 1). Not a non-sequitur, the clinical standing of analysis was the motivation, dictated from on high, for allowing psychoanalysts to continue working at the institute after Carl Müller-Braunschweig's letter to Anna Freud was intercepted by the Gestapo. In it he renewed his vows of loyalty to psychoanalysis as his higher power. And then there was Rittmeister's arrest and execution for high treason.

During the first phase of restructuring, the analytic "working group" was still assigned the letter A. Even the second round of restrictions put analysts in charge of catamnestic study, a research mode of follow-up evaluation of the clinical results of treatment, which decades later would be pressed into the service of obtaining insurance coverage for analytic and therapeutic treatment. Until the end of the Third Reich (or the destruction of the institute at the close of the war) the members of the Göring Institute could still check out books by Freud, which were kept in a special locked bookcase nicknamed by the insiders "the poison cabinet."

Rittmeister's introductory lecture at the Göring Institute carrying forward the reunification of all that took their departure from Freud is of the highest caliber, but the triad of analytic psychotherapies in which he orients himself is a dated throwaway. When Frederick Kohner in his Gidget novels upholds in the teen girl's family background an analytic psychotherapy that mixes Freudian, Adlerian, and Jungian approaches, we know that his general knowledge of psychoanalysis hailed from his time in the Berlin film industry.[6]

Rittmeister was given to reflect on the coordinates of the experimental synthesis underway at the Göring Institute – in the latter half of the 1930s largely from a Freudian perspective, while in the first half from the vantage of giving Jung the advantage. Earlier he assigned Adlerian therapy the role of booster supplement associated with Jung (and Marx); later, he elevated it, unexplored and intact, inside the new humanism.

Notes

1 For *Nazi Psychoanalysis* I wrote a very long caption to the photograph of the members of the Göring Institute attending a lecture with a portrait of Hitler on the wall. But as we were going to press it was felt that only the first shorter paragraph should stay, in which I addressed the missing portrait of Freud that allegedly faced the other portrait in the lecture hall until it was taken down in 1938. In the second paragraph I went on to talk about the reconfiguration of the analysts at the institute following Rittmeister's execution in 1943. A result of the change was that 1943 was displaced upwards and that 1938 vanished. In my text the correct date stands, but in the spectacular place of this caption I was suddenly responsible for misinformation and sensationalism. 1938 is amazing enough. A subsequent fact check does suggest a different placement of the portraits. Felix Boehm writes in 1937 that the portraits were for a time hanging side by side: "An der Wand des Institutes hinge nun wieder das Bild Freuds; allerdings neben dem Bild des Führers, das er aufzuhängen gezwungen war" (cited in Peglau, 440).

2 Following his studies with Carl Jung, and while he was Gustav Bally's didactic analysand, his extramural activities as a leftwinger prompted the Swiss authorities to curtail his stay there. Did the legendary discretion of Central Europeans mean that the Germans were not advised that he was in effect banished from Switzerland? Rittmeister was from a good family and knew how to dismiss annoying people with boundary issues. His friend Werner Krauss, who was also under arrest, witnessed the easy superiority

of Rittmeister firing up and backfiring following an interrogation. When a guard noted that Rittmeister seemed to have lost his brown tan, his teint, he almost lost it when his prisoner noted that he had never been a fan of brown.

3 The independent medical psychologist J.H. Schultz, who saw psychoanalysis as the contemporary face/interface of psychotherapy, may also have influenced M. Göring.

4 John F. Rittmeister, "Die Psychotherapeutische Aufgabe und der neue Humanismus," *PSYCHE*, 22, 12 (1968). Page references are given in the text. Originally published in *Zeitschrift Psychiatrische en Neurologische Bladen*, 5 (Amsterdam 1936). To give some sense of the modern sensibility he thought he could bring to the therapeutic milieu in Nazi Berlin, consider the comp he gives during his discussion of Jung's collective unconscious: "'human pathos formulae' (A. Warburg)" (940).

5 W. Kemper, "John F. Rittmeister zum Gedächtnis," *PSYCHE*, 147–149; here: 148 col. 2. The subsequent references to the article are given in the text.

6 See my discussion of the Gidget oeuvre in the third volume of *Critique of Fantasy* (Santa Barbara: punctum books, 2020–2021).

Chapter 4

Gejungt[1]

While in Switzerland Rittmeister had undergone and then come out of a fascination with Jung. The first act was documented in his 1930 review essay, "C.G. Jungs Energetik der Seele" (C.G. Jung's Energetics of the Soul), which welcomed Jung's opening wide of psychic reality over and against the close quarters of Freud's science.[2] Freud's earlier intervention in the "reductive materialist medical establishment" (17 col. 2), namely his emphasis on the individual psyche, got stuck in the one-sidedness to which drive theory led him. Jung argues that a subsuming or greater psychology can alone save Freudian psychoanalysis from a certain "decoding monotony" (17 col. 2). The second act of his Jung relationship, his disenchanted withdrawal from his former fascination, led to Rittmeister being regularly identified in the literature on the Göring Institute as an ex-Jungian.

That Jung historicized Freud's notion of the polymorphous organization of sexual instincts, as Rittmeister observes in 1930, was typical thinking for the times back then. Along these lines, then, Jung early on recommended Adler's dedication to the will to power as the enriching supplement to Freud's program (17 col. 2).

> It must be demonstrated that cultural formation is not only a surrogate, a sublimation, not just a substitute for the underlying motivating sexual substances, but rather that under certain conditions the "spiritual principle" (whatever that may be) is a principle sui generis that asserts itself with unheard-of power against that which is merely natural. (17 col. 2)

Rittmeister chooses the example of "homosexuality or incest love" to turn up the contrast between Freud and Jung. The former, a "causalist," would identify an "act of regression promoted by faulty development," while the latter, an "energist," would refrain from always speaking of perversion when faced with what might also be a necessary (even though transitional) phase of development, "which tends toward completely other, for example spiritual goals. Facts become here, one might say, symbols, since everything is conceived as being in flux" (17 col. 2).

Through his interpretation of dreams, Freud was the first to emplace the somatic inside the psychic. But Jung goes further (20 cols. 1–2). If Freud decodes dreams within an allegorical grid that yields the significance of the dreamer's relationality

DOI: 10.4324/9781003797708-6

to and in his world, then Jung's insistence that everything in the dream refers to and even communicates only with the dreamer, issuing warnings, offering guidance in taking the next step toward a higher consciousness, we encounter another reality only loosely attached to the object.

> This step in Jung's conception is extremely important in that so much that seemed up to this point to belong to the outer world must be recognized as belonging to interiority. If one can admit all that is projected into the outer world, one frees oneself from a good measure of primitivism or infantilism and serves the "reality principle," which indeed represents a major accomplishment. To measure (for instance) the value of this process one need only observe how strong the resistance of a neurotic is to letting go of projections, and in the big picture, as we experienced it for instance in the world war, the impact of general projections, of their grotesque misrepresentations of the contemporary world picture. (20 col. 2)

The positive recounting of Jung's innovative departures from Freud went down for a recount in Rittmeister's estimation around the time he joined the Berlin psychotherapy institute. Not published until long after his death, "Voraussetzungen und Konsequenzen der Jungschen Archetypenlehre" (Preconditions and Consequences of the Jungian Doctrine of Archetypes), is Rittmeister's openly political reckoning with Jung's figurehead role in the new culture of eclectic psychotherapy.[3]

> In the holy crusade against the science of destructive analysis, against the Devil of life-killing reason, C.G. Jung surprisingly quickly and with an elegant leap [*Sprunge*] also found himself under the stage lights of the political theater. There was no time to lose: one had long awaited him at the front of combat on behalf of the German world psyche. (1032)

Rittmeister drops his acerbic tone and turns to two failed dialectician couples, reminding the reader that Marx tried to go with Hegel before the couple split up – just as Jung went with the older Freud until the youngster reached a turning point of no return. Though Marx had to put Hegel back on his feet to advance the dialectic toward the present reality of sociology and history, Hegel the idealist was at least objective and included the beginnings of a very instructive realism. That doesn't apply to what Freud opened, the instinctual world of the individual. While never departing from the format of the individual, he thoroughly illuminated the process of development, which he tracked and propelled toward integration. "In the Oedipus complex he believed he found the image of the immanent dialectic of the decisive years of early childhood, which are at the same time the mythic early years of mankind" (1033).

Turning to the psyche of the schizophrenic, Jung discovered the fundamental proclivities for and products of fantasy. Forms of life, Jung decided, "could not be explained through the tragicomedies of the nursery and the destinies of the sexual instincts" (1033). He acknowledged instead that the

> dialectical principle with all its possibilities for constellation can emerge in man in countless forms, immersed in images presented in fantasy, art, dream and in symbols, which do not appear to stem from the individual infantile life but to be rather the late inheritance of phylogenetic existence. (1034)

Rittmeister questions the factor of inheritance in the Jungian dialectic. Polarities, admittedly a profound part of the whole organization of the human, are formed each time anew through regular interchange with the outer world and during a process of differentiation. "Man is like the whole of nature dialectically in motion between polar extremes, but this polarity is immanent not pre-existent and *is* in fact the mode of the course of all life, thought, and being itself" (1035). To underscore that all archetypes are links subsumed without exception by dialectical movement, Rittmeister quotes Lenin, who argued that science and technology, like the life histories of flora, fauna and mankind, impress upon man's brain not the idea of movement alone but the idea of movement returning to its starting point, i.e., dialectical movement. Rittmeister summons Lenin's assistance because Jung, although the placeholder of Marx in his conceit of twinned thinkers, is stuck like German fascism in the perspective of romantic idealism, which reached a dead end one hundred years ago.

Rittmeister cites Jung citing chapter and verse of separation of church and state – giving separately to God and to Caesar – to give form to the surrender of his thought. Rittmeister can now identify the God that entered Jungian subjectivity: "It is the God of the bourgeois order, of its state, its laws, which guarantee the philistine and the capitalist a pilgrimage of their own" [or: "unto themselves"] (1035). "For Jung, not only the external world but even God has slid down into subjectivity. The world of archetypes, the autonomous complexes, receive the attribute 'divine' and one of these (the self) is 'God in us'" (1035). It's at once a collective God and in its unity with the dark side "will no doubt one day reveal itself or has already revealed itself to be the folk community [*Volksgemeinschaft*] of exploiters, police, and workers" (1039).

The bourgeois forgoes comprehending the reasons and links underlying the crisis although the pressing sociological event demands a response. Instead, formerly veiled idealism becomes militant and instrumentalizes means of understanding the shadowy outer world like belief, intuition and empathy. The issues in history and sociology that also arise the bourgeois "cannot and must not see or want to see" (1039).

Notes

1 Gerhart Scheunert used "gejungt" in a postwar interview to characterize in part the synthesis that psychoanalysis was expected to undergo at the Göring Institute. It highlights a Jungian tilt in the resulting affectation, which is moreover verbified, as often happens in a faux formulation that ridicules. Scheunert signals with the past participial "gejungt" disparagement of the eclecticism his work followed out at that time, although

blaming Jung hardly characterizes its extent or nature. Moreover, for all his symptomatic acceptance of the opportunities that Nazi Germany afforded, Jung was hardly the sole mastermind behind the malaise that psychoanalysis endured in Nazi Germany. The case of Scheunert is a mainstay of my follow-up study (also with Routledge): *The Psychoanalysis of Nazism*.

2 John Rittmeister, "C.G. Jungs Energetik und Seele," *Ärztliche Rundschau*, 40 (1930), 17–20. Page references are given in the text.

3 John Rittmeister, "Vorraussetzungen und Konsequenzen der Jungschen Archetypenlehre," *PSYCHE*, 36, 11 (1982), 1032–1044. Page references are given in the text.

Chapter 5

Into the Frying Pan

Nowhere does Rittmeister's commitment to Marxism, which was real, spell out a comprehension as profound as that which he demonstrated regarding Freud and Jung. Rittmeister was not alone in being blocked from understanding analysis on the same page as Marxist sociology. His new humanism that emerged out of and alongside the polarization between Freud and Jung is the placeholder for this same page. Unnamed and readjusted, Adlerian therapy percolates up from the mix, mess and miss between the other two. It's also a vague waving through of what's in the foreground of Rittmeister's posthumous publications, the Marxism in the makeup of Adlerian therapy, which Matthias Göring of course did not acknowledge. A new humanism fronts for the unnameable third element going into the overcoming of the faceoff between Freud and Jung.

In his job talk Rittmeister argued that a humanistic approach belonging to this world is the bottom line that Freud already outlined. But a "new" humanism can no longer be as abstract as the old guy's version. Its novelty is Rittmeister's occasion for styling with the ideology of fitness to make his pitch. "If the suffering individual has fully experienced in himself the ugly and crooked refusals and blunders of life, then he will now... close ranks with those (*in die Truppen derjenigen einreihen*) who do not resign themselves meekly and weakly..., but instead he will learn to embody the will to change the world" (952).

The real freedom that the modern scientific-therapeutic pursuit of happiness can bring about in the here and now will not be restricted to private individuals (952–953).

> The psychotherapist treats persons who, not knowing the reason why, have fallen outside their individual and social possibilities. He addresses them, just as they address themselves in their isolation, at first as individuals and, by breaching their psychic armor, their illusions, restores the repressed drive power and renders the external world once more plausible. (951)

Childhood complexes and figures from the collective unconscious are divergent anthropological perspectives on the same point of departure, which Rittmeister situates in proximity to the psychotic state. The break with reality adjustment at the outer

DOI: 10.4324/9781003797708-7

limit of wish fantasy signals new worlds of psychotic delusion illuminated, however, by endopsychic insight. Jung, who recommended Daniel Paul Schreber's memoirs to Freud for close reading, resolutely indwelled this endopsychic affinity. "Just as the world of the schizophrenic is in fact the fantasized, hallucinated world, so the real world for the Jungian school signifies what has always been, the archetypal. This world is *wirklich*, real, *weil sie wirkt*, because it works, producing real effects" (943). While Rittmeister allows that interrogation of these effects for their truth content might seem as pointless as attempting to explain away an artist's figuration (943), to stop here, with Jung, just the same amounts to omitting human agency or activity, indeed, the very future of historical mankind (944). The usefulness of Freudian psychoanalysis in debunking deceptive rationalizations and empty ideals must, in turn, find application and illuminate the lawfulness and regularity of areas heretofore outside the ken of practical understanding and application (952).

Jung's system aims at unity: the healing of the terrible two of self-division. To be other, according to this system, is to be fallen, throwaway, trash (945). But Rittmeister counters, do not the schisms and tensions that Jung admits indicate instead that being other constitutes itself as activity and as part of the object world? Interiority has the innate tendency to get over itself beside itself and relate, after all, to reality (946). Here Rittmeister cites Daniel Paul Schreber as the proof at the limit that the reality of the others will be admitted. Rittmeister summons Schreber's acceptance of the separate reality of his fellow men, whom he had seen during his breakdown exclusively as miraculated up figures, to exemplify the inevitable leap out of the pre-logical mythical realm. On this leap Rittmeister would base the new humanism that must do for the community or for society what psychoanalysis achieved for the individual – a face to face with human suffering that does not make recourse to metaphysical or metaphorical comforts, whether as resigned acceptance or via aestheticization. "Modern scientific psychotherapy, similar to tendencies in political experiments, attempts to reclaim the place of nearly all that the European spirit has developed to date in the way of individual or collective systems in order to deal rigorously with such an allegedly divinely caused or naturally necessary tragedy" (935). These attempts are the moments of leaping, according to Rittmeister, or rather their running start following immersion of the infinite or eternal in finitude. "Since man as member of the human race potentially harbors the complete truth without however being able to realize it at once within his spatio-temporal limits, he is only able on occasion in ecstasy to leap toward a virtual totality" (948).

In his address to the Estates General of Psychoanalysis meeting in Paris in 2000, which through Major's influence was party to another attempt to promote Besserman Vianna's reckoning with the Lobo-Cabernite Affair, Derrida unwittingly cites or summons the discourse omitted from the transgenerational reading. After crediting psychoanalysis as the first discourse or institution to face human suffering without recourse to alibis he conjures with a leap a point beyond psychoanalysis to which psychoanalysis must aspire to reach outside itself and, accompanied by its special knowledge, realize an ethics, even a politics of psychoanalysis.

While Besserman Vianna and Major strongly suggest – if only because the three-generation reading requires it – that Kemper was involved in Rittmeister's arrest or at least didn't try to warn his colleague and analysand, there is no support for this allegation in the historical and transferential records. Christine Teller, the editor of Rittmeister's prison diaries,[1] argues that through the auto-analysis in his cell Rittmeister sought to continue his training analysis with Kemper (8). As Rittmeister entered in his diary: "I hope for so much from Kemper. That he will bring both the Gestapo and Göring to understand me and my fundamental innocence" (56). In his farewell letter to his brother Wolfgang (dated May 13, 1943) John recommends resources for understanding his fate: "You will learn quite a lot about me from Pastor Poelchen and it should make it easier for you to understand so much more, also please approach Dr. Kemper, who knows me and my complicatednesses (*Kompliziertheiten*) so precisely."[2]

In the prison diaries, Rittmeister views the momentum of his personal pattern of misfiring or backfiring attempts at progress since 1938 both in his private life and in his career as building toward a crisis for which his arrest and imprisonment were but the outward expression. His political involvements were, then, the very measure of the self-dissatisfaction he was seeking to escape. Rittmeister identifies the recent seminar he offered at the institute on mythology and schizophrenia and the research project on Descartes' mystical crisis, preliminary results of which he presented at the institute in 1942, as being symptomatically in sync with pressures building inside and out for which prison was the fitting container (53). In the paper he presented at the institute,[3] Rittmeister puts the case of Descartes on this line:

> Without a doubt Descartes was haunted by invasions from his unconscious, which had been in preparation for some time, but which now peaked, overwhelming him at this crisis point, at first irrationally, groundlessly. Instinctively he sought out solitude, withdrew into his poèle and, so to speak, hatched his interiority in the warmth of the philosophical fire. Similar to lone travellers by sea, who, as is well known, readily suffer hallucinations, so with Descartes, parallel to the diminished contact with the external world and his fellow man, the long averted side inside him became increasingly activated, so much so that strange phantoms appeared, and he was induced in a vision to turn around several times standing on his left foot, his left side having become independent and the right side of his body weak, "pirouetting" in the manner familiar to us from the circus ring [the word used can also signify the ward]. (214)

Long caught in the act of deciding between the alternatives of depression or neurosis and the sanity of conformity, Descartes was able through his crisis to find another way, one that bordered on the madness that he risked and which he took as his restarting point. He discovered, in Rittmeister's formulation, "ego as the Archimedean point from which the world can be animated" (218). He thus also recognized nature as a field of inquiry, a maternal aspect and reckoning that can be seen to underlie the nine years he waited before giving a publishable body to the insights that emerged during the night of crisis. At the interchange between nine years and nine months Rittmeister drops a footnote to Freud's study of demonological neurosis. The footnote was presumably silent when Rittmeister presented his Descartes reading in 1942. Its restoration and indeed the publication of Rittmeister's text we owe to Kemper, who urged reprinting Rittmeister's most important essays by 1973, the 30-year anniversary of his death date.

The poèle (oven, stove or frying pan) in the small encampment where Descartes spent his night of crisis and breakthrough is a recurring image and reference throughout Rittmeister's prison diaries. As is made clear in entries addressed "ad Kemper," it was moreover a transference prop or signal exchanged within the didactic analytic relationship. It seems evident that both hoped that they would succeed in constructing Rittmeister's political activities as acting outs along a psychopathological continuum. Thus, the arrest would be seen to serve a therapeutic purpose and, in Rittmeister's case of political aberration, the prognosis for a subject of good stock would be considered excellent. Through psychotherapy, including the extolled therapeutic correctness of the Nazi regime, Rittmeister would be saved for psychotherapy – conceived as one of the foundations of the newly discovered and applied psychologization of the socius at war.

It seems that just about every move analytic therapy made in Nazi Germany took a 50-50 risk. The course of the war could tip the scales. "Who knows whether there might not be an early amnesty. Just now the crisis in the war is unmistakable" (86). Rittmeister appears to suggest or hope that the time of crisis still allowed for a 50-50 chance. Would the change for the better that analytic psychotherapy had proved capable of bringing about allow him a second chance or would he meet with the dead set determination waiting in the right wings of the corridors of German science to eliminate the potential contaminant of degeneracy.

Following his arrest in 1942, Rittmeister was covered by colleague Harald Schultz-Hencke, whose latest book *Der gehemmte Mensch* (The Inhibited Man) he was reading very closely during his imprisonment, taking it as the frame for his future rehabilitation and thus also, he underscored in the asides addressed to Kemper, as the model for how he should be and should have been analyzed. He establishes a continuity shot between his own placement in charge of the clinic in lieu of the Freudians Boehm and Müller-Braunschweig and the revisionist inroad that his replacement by Schultz-Hencke represented. But after Rittmeister's absence was made permanent, Werner Kemper, whose training placed him among the Freudians, was made the director of the clinic in 1943. Schultz-Hencke's first wife was non-Aryan and so he couldn't hold the position of director beyond the interim stint. Kemper and Schultz-Hencke remained collegial, and their postwar affinity, since Kemper was soon living and working in Brazil, never had to be put to the test.

In the transferential sidelines of his reading of his successor's new book, Rittmeister was concerned that his training analyst had been viewing him much too optimistically, indeed just as he sees himself from the vantage of only one of his sides (92). Translation: Kemper liked Rittmeister too much. In the diary entries marked "ad Kemper," Rittmeister constructs his analysis as overly concerned with intimacy issues, including sexual difficulties, and unwilling to intervene in and interrupt neurotic patterns with a directive word from the sponsor (90–91). Rittmeister enters in his prison journal on November 21, 1942:

> In the first place I must remain aware that things just couldn't continue as they were before the arrest. My reading of Schultz-Hencke's *Inhibited Man* has helped me to see this clearly. Something had to happen; if not the arrest, then I would have entered a severe crisis, or, as so often before, a period of apathy and dragged myself along. (92)

From his prison diaries, Rittmeister looked back upon his crisis, growing on him since 1938, as bordering on psychosis but which the cell therapy initiated by his arrest had doubled and contained. His cell time administers the *Gegengift* (antidote) against his earlier depression (56) and "engenders at once the highest stimulus to live" (68). "At the same time, I must keep in mind that the way my life was in August/September, so lethargic and without impulse, could not have continued. An intervention had to follow!" (68). And it did and he now reaps or reads the benefits. "But the plasticity, the treasure, the connection with the whole grows, the more my situation becomes a threat: then the quotations from Schopenhauer or from the New Testament also grow luminous" (61). "Noteworthy items that no analysis would have manifested now emerge" (71). Can the enormity of his new feeling for life continue after the imprisonment? Only upon containment, collecting oneself in a tight spot, can one go deep. "But the will to encompass everything of import is hard to eradicate. That is the source of melancholia" (72).

In prison, then, he began to return to life's affirmational metabolism – and he looked forward to the necessary post-prison work of his stabilization, sustaining his psychic gains during the incarceration on the outside in his life and work. "The rigor of daily demands and the anxious armoring forced me to wear masks" (79). Now he experiences his own vulnerability, his need for a guardian angel.

Rittmeister analyzed himself in diary entries addressed not only to Kemper but also to the authorities, whom he had to convince that his political activity was a treatable neurosis that could be sloughed off his well-stocked professional persona. His work running the clinic was praiseworthy. Perhaps to underscore his professional contribution he also wrote in jail a scientific essay in dialogue form: "Moral in Stufenfolgen" ("Morality in a Sequence of Steps").[4] The editors of the posthumous publication acknowledge Kemper as their source. Rittmeister scribbled the fragment on packing paper in his cell, and the prison chaplain preserved it following Rittmeister's execution. He gave the fragment to the widow, Eva Rittmeister, upon her release from imprisonment. The editors, in concert no doubt with those who safeguarded and transmitted the text, ascribe to Renatus, Jordanus and Johannes, the interlocutors in the three-way conversation, the keyed-in signatories, respectively, Descartes, Giordano Bruno and Marx. It's very likely that Rittmeister invited the interlocutors to be identified most readily – and given the work of reunification of psychoanalysis with the breakaway analytic therapies that brought him to Berlin and to this impasse – with the monikers (in the same order) Freud, Jung and Adler.

In the diaries Rittmeister spells out that he first became acquainted with Marx's thought on a "Jungian basis" (105). That basis or bottom line survived his disaffection with Jungian mysticism: "I was still drawn to nondifferentiated becoming, but in the real world rather than in connoisseur contemplation and projection of past cults and Far-Eastern cultures. For it was here that the world burned" (41).

In the prison dialogue, he subsumes his Marxism as political infraction, in theory and therapy, within the *Bildungsroman* of the psychotherapies finding a more perfect union in Nazi Germany. The first figure or position underscores attainment of autonomy over and against blind belief by taking the driving seat from the unconscious (which becomes more audible as backseat driver). One must, however, not remain stuck in natural uninhibited being. This step away from the naïve and natural starting position is attended by suffering, isolation, and finding oneself in possession of a will of one's own. "Reunification" names the third step. One turns again to the world but from a higher vantage point. "One is self but still member of the whole" (150 col. 1). A balance in becoming is achieved: normal egotism or pursuit of happiness is the goal. This brings us to Jordanus, the Jung position.

What lies beyond the pursuit of happiness is disclosure of insight into profound – metaphysical, cosmic – connections. Rittmeister lists the three character-types thus disposed. There is the sensitive individual, who is "schizoid" to a problematic degree, in whom "incorrigibly inhibited and nevertheless effective expansions lead to ambivalence, contradiction etc." (150 col. 1). The next type is the "contemplative-introverted" individual, whose "relations with the outside world are reduced through repression." This one's leading themes are "inner life, thinking, brooding, alienation from nature and immediacy" (150 col. 1). The third type is a crowd: "Finally those afflicted with great suffering, having gone from valuation of the outer world to investment in the interior, now experience the opposed pairs: world – interiority, happiness – denial etc." (150 col. 1). For all three types, the "inner split is unbridgeable," fundamental or "inborn-immanent" (150 col. 1).

While Jung considers, in English in the original, "the split in the libido" to be an anthropological condition rather than a consequence of the dynamic of repression, Freud and Schultz-Hencke "assume a certain degree of repression to be ubiquitous" (151 col. 1). The first type of illness is at the same time the Cartesian or Freudian illness. The second mode of affliction is the position of Bruno or Jung conceived at once as illness and as interpretation of illness:

> What is considered at the first level as error, that is, as illness, becomes here world destiny and fall from the whole (God), eternal guilt etc. The individual complexes (father, mother, love, hate, castration etc.) correspond to pre-formed primal images (archetypes); the individual process of development [*Bildungsprozeß*] is displaced onto divine or natural principles, in which one participates. (151 col. 1)

While Rittmeister continues to develop the revalorization, he brings it all to the catastrophe of psychosis, the turning point that brings up the case of Schreber. Many individuals take it all only ideally and fail to accept the consequence of "reaching the reality of the other" (151 col. 1). The only way to save this level or step is to integrate it within the next level, that of Johannes (or Marx or Adler). Here we step over the pathological consequences of development, one of which introjects a Schreber quotation:

> My fellow men, for whom there was still no consideration, are neither raw material for my expansion ("élargissement du moi") nor illusion ("quickly improvised men") but rather are equal to me in my essence. Steps I (autonomy) and II (surrender to the world as a whole), which can interpenetrate one another, attain their character of moving beyond the ego only if I again become real and in praxis take as life's maxim the support of the well-being of the others (social welfare). Only in this way can the lonely ego receive a sense for the value of life. (151 col. 2)

In taking the third step, the psyche returns to reality at a higher but more practical level.

Notes

1 John Rittmeister, *"Hier brennt doch die Welt." Aufzeichnungen aus dem Gefängnis 1942–1943 u.a. Schriften* ("Here the World is Burning." Notes from Prison 1942–1943 Among Other Writings), ed. Christine Teller (Gütersloh: Verlag Jakob van Hoddi, 1992). Page references are given in the text.

2 Walter Bräutigam, *John Rittmeister – Leben und Sterben* (Living and Dying) (Ebenhausen bei München: Langewiesche-Brandt Verlag, 1999), 42. Pastors Poelchen and Ohm visited Rittmeister regularly in prison.

3 J. Rittmeister, "Die mystische Krise des jungen Descartes" (The Mystical Crisis of Descartes as a Young Man), *Zeitschrfit für Psychosomatische Medizin und Psychoanalyse*, 15, 3 (1969), 204–224. Page references are given in the text. Apparently, Matthias Göring was able to brace himself in the face of Rittmeister's arrest for treason because he found the presentation on Descartes so suspect.

4 John Rittmeister, "Moral in Stufenfolgen (als Gespräch auszuarbeiten)," *Zeitschrift für Psychosomatische Medizin und Psychoanalyse* 14, 2 (1968), 150–152. Page numbers are given in the text.

Chapter 6

Captive Analysis and the Specifics of the Transference

Kemper's 1968 eulogy draws on what he learned of Rittmeister's history in session, a family history befitting a Thomas Mann narrative:[1]

> The discrepancy of the blood of his Huguenotte, English, and Dutch ancestors, the traditional ties of a senator's family from Hamburg on his mother's side, the worldwide expansion of the father's overseas company, the grand style of the family home, a late flowering of the concluding Victorian era, and in addition the birth of a twin-sibling-couple (*eines Zwillingsgeschwisterpärchens*) when he was one and a half – all that and more had to be worked through inwardly and brought into an attempted harmony and had a strong impact on his character. (147 col. 1 – col. 2)

The key term in the history Kemper takes is the couple of twins, brother and sister. Brother Wolfgang spent long periods of time away from the family situation, leaving the way open for his older brother to glom onto his twin sister Edith. This "little couple" was for Rittmeister, then, an internal simulacrum of the primal scene which he entertained or which entertained him at the other's peril.

The import of Luigi Pirandello's *Six Characters in Search of an Author*, the first intertext in Rittmeister's prison reflections and memoirs, is that he attended a performance with Edith (32) and that it became the inspiration for his intellectual pursuits. "The study of this authentic reality would later become my guideline [*Leitlinie*] (psychoanalysis, sociology)" (33).

In Pirandello's play,[2] life is comprised of absurdities that don't need to be credible since they're true, while theatre (i.e., Oedipus) imposes a mold of credibility to give the appearance of truth. Life's drama or trauma broke this mold (10). The spokesman for the characters is FATHER whose multi-perspectival reflection on their state – "Each one of us is lots and lots of people" (26) – is grounded in responsibility and guilt. The father was possessed, as his SON mockingly puts it, by a "Daemon of Experiment" (17). All the harm, in short, resulted from his efforts to do good (20).

The characters don't inhabit the suffer zone of a changing reality, which the actors and the director traverse via illusion. The characters "don't exist outside this illusion" (55), a realm that is for them unchanging (11). Parts of an author in a

DOI: 10.4324/9781003797708-8

state of unintegration, the characters belong to a realm of the mothers but under the aegis of trauma. MOTHER is against showing the scene or wound. It's in the past, the director responds. But for her the scene can't be delivered lest she be delivered of the scene. We encounter here the prospect of a traumatic responsibility. "No, it's happening now! It's happening all the time! … I'm alive and it's alive and it keeps coming back again and again, as fresh as the first time." Everything, everyone in the closed circuit or loop of the characters stuck on two or three scenes is there to keep her agony going, going, but never gone (52).

The riveting trauma with its "immutable reality" (58) unfolds as scenes for characters an author conceived but didn't deliver, scenes for the not fully born which are fantasies, each more primitive than the last, each belonging to a phase earlier than the last. The first scene turns on adult father/daughter incest, the next rebounds within the Oedipal triangle, and the final scene takes regression to the pre-Oedipal stage. Between two siblings in childhood there's murder by death wish (the drowned little girl) followed by suicide (the boy). The corpse of the boy who shoots himself for real is the bottom line that the stepdaughter from the incest scene can step over, exiting the theater laughing.

The author created the characters, gave them life, but didn't bring them to birth in life, so they can't die (12–13). He also didn't bring them to death in life. Pirandello's presentation of a sibling *Liebestod* in a milieu of unfinished birth filling the precincts of pre-Oedipal mother and infant merger before which the father of incest stands guard is a diagnostic guide to the retrofitting of the unconscious in adaptation to modern European history in the making. Rittmeister selects it as his souvenir of the failure of incest to find a home on the stage of life. The drama's ongoing performance of a stricken family system subsuming authorship swabbed over into the audience where Rittmeister was sitting with his sister. *Six Characters in Search of an Author*, which premiered in 1921, belongs to the period of upheavals in Italy that led to Mussolini's dictatorship, setting the search for authority on a family system in crisis. Psychoanalysis sees through the family life that only struts the stage – but is unable to put it back together again.

Rittmeister went to Italy with Edith trying to lift her spirits. They participated in the first anniversary celebrations of the 1922 fascist march on Rome. She was out of one engagement and into another unhappy relationship. When he finds that he is making little progress in his attempt to lift his sister's severe depression, he takes her to Berlin to see his former analytic therapist, Hans von Hattingberg. "Hattingberg however was living then in a very extraverted way with a new wife" (36). After an engaging evening with von Hattingberg in the circle of his artist friends, Edith killed herself. The way was open now for Rittmeister's first "exogamous" girlfriend. His piano playing (given, as analysis knows best, in memoriam of masturbation in early childhood) is the still open connection to Edith (33).

His sister Edith withdrew just as Rittmeister was able to begin to approach her. It was this way with his mother, too. Both women offered the counterweight to the alienated relationship to father. "These real losses (mother and Edith) were unconsciously perhaps only confirmations of the loss of love in childhood" (36).

On her death bed the mother exacted the father's promise to let the son pursue his scholarly and scientific inclinations rather than become another merchant (33). That was in 1919, the year she died of the breast cancer diagnosed at the start of the war (29). He trained for the war effort as a *Funker* (radio operator) and served as an extra in propaganda films. At the time of writing the diary in prison he lists his five top interests: number three is *Flugzeugbau* (aircraft construction) (21). He prefers the culture of the south, a hotbed of his family romance fantasies from which he was cut off at the kitchen, "where everything originates," which was off limits (25). The household *Schmutzkomplex* (mysophobia) kept him from the tender and tellurian aspects of mother (25). While the first fact of his life was oral disappointment at the mother's breast – to get him to start sucking baby John had to be tapped on the cheeks (19) – the timing of the complex under construction in the prison diaries begins during latency, for example with his flat chest, which played a role in his hypochondriacal imaginings (20). Again, he writes that the two women who died on him confirmed the reservations indelibly introduced by the loss of paternal love ("väterliche Liebesverlust") at age six (25).[3]

Rittmeister shifts out of the topography of schizophrenia and suicide marked by family and friends toward the treatable terrain of the homosexuality neurosis indwelling his heterosexuality. In 1923, he began acquiring "the first appetite for women" (39). When he first met the woman he would wed, she was dressed for the ball like a boy (51). The woman who wants to be an actress (53) goes by the nickname Mackie, which carries "the knife." If they could only have had a child, he laments, then one thing would have led to another, like with the Kemper couple (56).[4] Later on he returns to the saving prospect of children, only to allow that his fatherhood now would be a confidence game; only once his deneuroticization is further along could he truly be a father (91). Rittmeister fits the profile of the German intellectual or artist, who from Goethe to Thomas Mann is a fragile blend served straight up with a twist. At the start of his prison diaries, he takes his own history. A neurotic disposition is guaranteed by a constitutional and psychic change at age nine or ten (19–20). No longer pretty, he was overwhelmed by feelings of inferiority and anxiety. This is related to a loss or withdrawal of paternal love (25). As a little philosopher he was cute.

> Fear of growing older was very central. The basic complex was: if only it would be the way it was in the first ten years, and who proved unfaithful and to whom is my hate-love addressed? Father (do the effects of this continue to this day?). (33)

The psychosomatic syndication of his troubles – heart pains and blushing – commences in high school (*Gymnasium*). He picked up on "a stream of erotic seduction" emanating from his Latin instructor. His learning was inhibited; he couldn't concentrate; he blushed and batted his eyes (and battled these tics) whenever the instructor stood behind him during extemporaneous translation exercises. He never acquired a foundation in Latin. His ability to play freely or wildly with the fisher boys was inhibited, both in fact and in fantasy (21). "Burst openings and explosive bits made me difficult to raise or educate. – Looking back longingly on the uninhibited life ('the blonde-haired and blue-eyed,' see *Tonio Kröger*), I nevertheless had to take the prescribed intellectual and contemplative path of the unnaive" (28). All the while wrapping the "onion layers" around his true self or ego he was suppressing sexual feeling (30). "Rigidly a sort of armor was maintained until the first analysis in 1922, when, for the first time, anxiety became conscious" (30).

As noted, Rittmeister's first analysis was with Hans von Hattingberg, whose association with the Göring Institute was in connection with the research project on homosexuality. In his 1936 study *Über die Liebe. Eine ärztliche Wegweisung* (On Love. A Medical Guide) he cosigned the consensus highlighting the neurosis in homosexuality.[5] He opens the section on "The Samers" (*Die Gleichlinge*) by invoking the faux insider's view, fashionable in Weimar Germany, that homosexuality is a third gender simply not at home to heterosexuality (65). After taking the usual tour of the homosexual greats of history, von Hattingberg changes direction: "Here homosexuality will be treated as a particular position in love, as a specific method to deal with the difficulties associated with love. For the physician homosexuality thus comes to occupy a place next to neurosis, which is the typical attempted solution of problems that life in the community presents to man" (65). We could walk down another hall of fame in which many neurotics would stand tall as accomplished individuals.

According to analytic sexology homosexuality is the normal intermediary phase between narcissism and heterosexuality (70). Even though, he argues, the observed lack of such a phase in too many cases has by now invalidated this model, two aspects continue to be right on. The attraction to one's own sex alone cannot be considered perverse. And the only thing wrong about masturbation is that there can be a withdrawal from contact. The convenience stories of *Notonanie* (expedient masturbation) and the *Auch-Homosexuellen* (the also homosexuals) don't veto a developing heterosexual identity (51, 78). Add to the isolating trend in masturbation the "mechanism" of sexualization, which turns types of anxiety, for example, into sexual excitement (63), and we have the basics of all perversion: "We find here the essential trait of all inversion: the exclusion of human *Berührung* (contact, physical touch, nearness) and the extraction of pleasure out of the tension of distance" (82). As set forth by analytic sexology, the sequence of phases rings true to von Hattingberg: there is a natural increase culminating in heterosexuality. For the introverted personality every turn of interest to another human being is already a step beyond. "The 'samer,' who doesn't go any further than to another of the same kind, remains stuck halfway; he doesn't make the decisive step toward the most other" (70).

Rittmeister developed a strong attachment to von Hattingberg, but then freed himself "in a wild altercation" in 1930 reproaching him for not analyzing his aggressive tendencies (35).[6] When Rittmeister tallies his own upcoming execution with the unnatural deaths of his father (who committed suicide in 1940) and Edith, also taking into account the unquiet death of his mother, he wonders what his brother Wolfgang, the sole survivor, will think "when he surveys the field of rubble of the family" (88). John's free to think it was for the best not to have children since it would seem there is an "unnatural kernel of destiny" in the family line, one best not to be continued. The reason he separated from his family was the *Grundgefühl* (basic feeling) that was long dominant, namely that there wasn't any point (24). "But now… I yearn for a simple life… away from the artificial cerebral existence" (24). Sixty pages later in the diary, with the inevitability of his execution upon him, his thoughts go out to his brother, and he knows that it is too late.[7]

Rittmeister records in his prison diaries dreams like exhibits in the treatable neurosis defense. The setting for the defense in Nazi Germany is a pervasive awareness and elaboration of homoerotic seductiveness matched by the absence of actual homosexuality. Instead, it's a neurotic tendency in Rittmeister or Tonio Kröger, for example, which like treason can be worked through. In the dream a sailor (whose description is highly charged) goes against what the dreamer anticipates when he doesn't pick up the small pretty girl standing by. The sailor splits and Rittmeister engages the girl instead in lively conversation (60). Following a dream in which he is about to drop his *Lederhosen* (62), another dream stages a terrific fight with J.H. Schultz. In the dream Rittmeister's highly successful independent colleague (that is, not identified as belonging to working group A, B or C) faults the dreamer's case presentations. He realizes that he's finished at the institute, a release from his duties Rittmeister notes must be related to his arrest (63).

The founder of autogenic training, which he introduced a year before the Nazi takeover, Schultz was active at the Berlin Institute in the treatment of homosexual patients, often soldiers who like the war neurotics were treated and not condemned. Schultz's assistant reported on a session she witnessed in which a patient performed his cure with a prostitute before a "jury" of experts. This snippet circulates widely but unaccompanied by any context, argument or supporting, corroborating evidence. Even Karen Brecht and co. included it as sufficient indictment of Schultz in their catalogue for the official return to Germany of international psychoanalysis, the 1985 Hamburg conference. But the fucker, getting off exhibiting himself to surrounding men in military uniforms, was saved as a result, admittedly only for as long as it would take to die in combat.

Notes

1 Werner Kemper, "John F. Rittmeister zum Gedähtnis," page references are given in the text.

2 Luigi Pirandello, *Six Characters in Search of an Author*, trans. Felicity Firth, in *Collected Plays*, ed. Robert Rietty, volume 2 (New York: Riverrun Press, 1988). Page references are given in the text.

3 Outside this homoerotic confessional tract in the prison writings, the Rittmeister father/son relationship stands out among the family histories of the Göring Institute members. On his own Rittmeister junior aided Jewish patients, even securing one woman's flight to Cuba as late as 1939 through his well-connected father in Hamburg. Walter Bräutigam, who came to the Göring Institute at the time of Rittmeister's arrest to train as a psychoanalyst, wrote both the afterword to Christine Teller's edition of Rittmeister's prison writings and a commemorative monograph, *John Rittmeister – Leben und Sterben* (Ebenhausen: Langewiesche-Brandt, 1987). Bräutigam documents Rittmeister's efforts on behalf of his Jewish patients in the former (175–176) as well as in the latter (31).

4 In 1968, following his divorce from his wife, Kemper elaborates the importance of Rittmeister's late marriage to a younger woman, as though responding to the captive author's sense of Kemper's model family situation. "A rich hitherto unknown fulfillment came to Rittmeister through his 1939 marriage. His young wife was for him the symbol of the happy realization of that which he himself had searched for all his life. Out of the teacher–student relationship arising from the age difference, a satisfying enriching partnership developed in lieu of his former aloneness" (149 col. 1). It doesn't sound like they needed to follow the lead of Kemper's marriage with children.

5 Hans von Hattingberg, *Über die Liebe. Eine ärztliche Wegweisung* (Munich: Kindler Verlag, 1975). Page references are given in the text.

6 Hans von Hattingberg was born in Vienna but set up shop in Munich in 1913. While he was interested in Freud's science and was a member of the Psychoanalytic Society in Vienna, I found no indication that he in fact was a psychoanalyst. In 1932 he relocated to Berlin and became affiliated there with the Institut für Psychologische Forschung und Psychotherapie, a good fit since already in the 1920s he was interested in the Adler, Jung, Freud triangle as the fulcrum for a new psychotherapy. He served at the Göring Institute as director of the research division (*Forschungsabteilung*). He died in Berlin in 1944. The second marriage, a change in milieu that Rittmeister and his sister found so off-putting, ended in divorce.

7 I consulted Peter Weiss's novel *The Aesthetics of Resistance* (Die Ästhetik des Widerstands) (Frankfurt a/M: Suhrkamp Verlag, 2005) for its excruciating reconstruction of the execution of the leading figures of the Red Orchestra following months of imprisonment, interrogation and torture. I had to take on the challenge of reading Weiss's thousand-page counter-Reich for the sole mention of John Rittmeister's execution. It's odd but perhaps on the mark that it leaves out psychoanalysis: "Rittmeister, the medical doctor and psychiatrist, had demonstrated through his death that for some time already the group of resisters was classless" (1148).

Part Two

Acquitting WK

Chapter 7

Happy Kemper

Was Werner Kemper following Rittmeister's lead in recognizing in the corpus of Schultz-Hencke what the future held in store, the future as extrapolated from his years at the Berlin Institute? Schultz-Hencke's work gave surety that there could be a happy medium for and continuity with the benign advances of Greater Psychoanalysis.[1] Were Kemper's postwar efforts on behalf of analytic psychotherapy in alliance with Harald Schultz-Hencke a response to Rittmeister's prison address to him, ad Kemper? Or was it a season of deferred obedience to the dictates of the Göring Institute? While the book he published in the Third Reich was so camouflaged or autocensored that even inside readers were hard pressed to recognize it as psychoanalytic, several presentations he gave at the institute, which were published after the war, are resolutely Freudian.

The two survivors, Kemper and Schultz-Hencke, set up shop again in the ruins, expressly saving the original Berlin psychoanalytic institute, which was the continuity shot passing through the Göring Institute. But their emphasis was placed, strange but true, on the work during the Nazi years resulting from cooperation with colleagues from the different schools. It seems the prospect of starting over in Brazil put a stop to Kemper's overvaluation of mixing it up with the psychotherapies.

Freud judged Schultz-Hencke the inner enemy of psychoanalysis in Berlin and warned adamantly against letting him take too much power in the wake of the clearing out of the Jews. The first time Schultz-Hencke taught at the psychoanalytic institute in 1927/1928 was the occasion for his exclusion from the teaching faculty – not only on account of his critique of the sexual theory but also because he advocated combining the concept of analysis with Adlerian and Jungian approaches. Already falling in line with something like the Göring Institute he was that much more slippery for not being at all Nazi.

In the 1939 preface to *Der gehemmte Mensch* (The Inhibited Man) Schultz-Hencke foregrounds his lexical innovations as crucial to the reestablishment of psychoanalytic theory based on a strictly professional scientific terminology. "Depth psychology" works with available words and thus its literature is accessible – or seemingly accessible – to a wide circle of readers. This access is more than what the taboos surrounding its topics should allow. But how can a science remain vital without the background support of a seriously interested and invested world of laymen? How

DOI: 10.4324/9781003797708-10

can its therapeutic aspect be dedicated to the good of mankind if only insiders can understand the discourse in which the therapy is embedded? A middle way must be found between esoteric science and the popularization of problematic findings. The entirety of the book, the author concludes, is the experimental attempt to find this middle path.

In the postwar preface (1946), Schultz-Hencke assures the readership that he hasn't made any alterations, though he would have liked to tone down the criticism of Freud and his school. In the meantime, the criticism dates his work: in England and even more so in America a mature assimilation of psychoanalytic findings is underway. Now the book can document what it was still possible to publish in the Third Reich in circumvention of the censorship. Any changes to his text would look like rote "adaptations" to the new situation. The only change he did introduce, however, was deletion of the subtitle and concept of "Desmolyse." Since scientific world opinion, Schultz-Hencke continues, has set aside Freud's outmoded sexual theory in addition to large portions of his so-called metapsychology it now appears gratuitous to improve the naming of concepts no longer current. In closing, he notes with satisfaction that a Neo-psychoanalytic working group (*Arbeitsgruppe*) has been formed in Berlin based on an amalgamation of the doctrines of Freud, Adler and Jung, just the kind of synthesis one can find already presented and accounted for in *Der gehemmte Mensch.*

Schultz-Hencke's approach to psychopathology, which was expressly inspired by Freud's 1896 article, "Further Remarks on the Neuro-Psychoses of Defense," counted the neurotic and the psychotic as at bottom the same patient with the same basic issues, whose symptomatology, however, reflected a different balance in the so-called simultaneity of organic or physical conditions and psychic etiology. He keeps the common ground of a united understanding of neurosis and psychosis as the preamble to the understanding and treatment of their singularities. His interpretations of the difficulties or inhibitions that both neurotics and psychotics symptomatize, only differently given the shifting balancing act of simultaneity between physical and psychic factors, doesn't so much minimize psychosis as reformat the general theory of psychic reality and interpersonal therapy for relating to and stabilizing psychosis.

His 1952 *Das Problem der Schizophrenie. Analytische Psychotherapie und Psychose* (The Problem of Schizophrenia. Analytic Psychotherapy and Psychosis) was the summum of his career. Dismissed by international reviewers as hardly new, the book that was to be his triumph proved a disappointment. Steering through the Bermuda triangle of the three depth psychologies may have inhibited international recognition of his Neo innovativeness given that the colleagues in the States had already embarked upon similar renovations but without all that dated material. Just the same, Schultz-Hencke's approach to treating psychotic patients was highly influential in both Germanies after the war. The author also plies, I think self-consciously, a certain affinity with Rittmeister's sensibility and language. Viewed from the shore of the norm, Schultz-Hencke writes, psychotic experience represents a *Sprung* ("leap" or "crack") (78). You must overlook the sensational aspects of psychotic experience, he clarifies, in contemplating its singular *Sprung*. Many readers who have followed up to this point, the author admits, may well, understandably, hesitate before making the "leap" into what is qualitatively a different kind of reality. At first contact, the psychotic presents aberrant phenomena that do not appear understandable along the lines of the psychology of neurosis. But the essential content of this study, Schultz-Hencke underscores, holds these appearances to be deceptive.

Most important for contextualizing Werner Kemper and John Rittmeister is that between *The Inhibited Man* and *The Problem of Schizophrenia* Schultz-Hencke belonged to the cozy corner in which Kemper resided with his dead friend. The outer supporting walls were erected post war. There is no indication other than Rittmeister's prison address that the senior colleague was particularly close to Kemper at the Göring Institute. Maybe they cooperated in the running of the clinic following Rittmeister's arrest. But it's only in the documentation of the immediate postwar period that we find an understanding between them in the parerga of the discourse of directives. Schultz-Hencke and Kemper became at once active collaborators in promoting analytic psychotherapy in Berlin and close friends. All the institute veterans were left doing the shuffle of trying to find a way to practice psychotherapy. Was it too late to draw a line differentiating analysis and therapy or were there simply too few analysts around to reconfigure psychoanalysis proper in Berlin right after 1945?

Many years later and back in Germany, Kemper, in his contribution to *Psychotherapie in Selbstdarstellungen* (Psychotherapy in Self-Presentations), again salvages the war years as positive influence on his development as therapist. "After the fact I experience these years as a time of clarification of my own position in the daily discussions with the likeminded and differently oriented colleagues."[2] These discussions were productive in the eclectic spirit of sorting through and selecting the best treatment techniques for a given case. "Instead of losing ourselves in the usual endless theoretical discussions about opposed positions which tend to remain sterile, we could here focus on the data of the concrete case and assess the pros and cons of every treatment modality" (278). His 1973 CV shores itself up with Freud, who, Kemper proudly notes, recommended one of his articles for publication in the international journal (279). But he also tucks into the corner acknowledgment of the contact he enjoyed with J.H. Schultz through their work at the institute's clinic (288).

Kemper sacrificed his reputation by making the move to Brazil or so it seemed upon his return. It's hard to judge what postwar prominence in Germany Kemper felt he was owed. In the "Self-Presentation," the stretch from Freud to J.H. Schultz is the niche in which he placed his memorial. But that honor roll is too skewed, too much of a reach for a personal claim to fame. Instead, he belabors his part played in history. And it was his restoration of the clinic in 1946 together with Schultz-Hencke that has historical import. The renewed clinic, Kemper underscores, made history by being the first to afford those without means free psychotherapeutic and psychoanalytic treatment (298). The professionalization of psychotherapy that was continued, indeed promoted in the Third Reich made next steps possible that would lead, one, to the integration in Germany of analytic psychotherapy in the medical profession and, two, to the categorical suitability of its treatment, which qualified for health insurance coverage.

After the history-making he engaged in with Schultz-Hencke, Kemper followed Jones's call to Brazil. Why doesn't he make the pitch for being the founding father of official psychoanalysis in Rio de Janeiro? At the time he composed this self-presentation his restraint cannot readily be explained by the crises and scandals that soon shook and later overtook his institute.[3]

Kemper had a knack for treating leading political figures. Matthias Göring's wife Erna was in analysis with him over the Nazi years, passing along information that he could use for his own sake and for the protection of others. It must have come as a surprise when she converted to Freudian analysis, even choosing to be educated and trained as a clinician in her own right. For years she had taken delight in terrorizing the analysts with her Heil Hitler greeting, which as always required an echoing response.

Was nothing about Rittmeister conveyed in this confessional? The possibility is the only kernel of reality in the suspicion that Kemper didn't warn Rittmeister. Surely Erna's husband would have realized by then, however, that his wife, who, like their son, too, was in training to become a psychoanalyst, was no longer his confidante. Kemper would have been especially careful about inviting any kind of exchange regarding Rittmeister, who, as he knew, hid Jews en route to escaping Germany at the Klinik Waldhaus, also helping them and others in their emigration journeys via his familial connections in Hamburg. No one seems to speculate on the repercussions of Kemper's confidential receipt of all this evidence of treason.[4]

Rittmeister's application for a visa to give lectures in Switzerland about his work at the Berlin clinic, planned for early May 1942, was suddenly revoked, which might well have signaled official awareness of Rittmeister's serious political infractions.[5] Kemper would have known about this setback. No doubt it could be ascribed to the turn for the worse in the Nazi war effort, which was experienced by the denizens of the citadel in fortress Europe as a battening down of all sorts of expectations and hopes.

In postwar Berlin Kemper was apparently treating a higher up who assured him that the divided city would be the frontline in the third war that was coming soon. He recalls in a booklet he devoted to his Brazil years: "For the sake of my children I was determined to start over again completely on my own."[6] The friendship with Schultz-Hencke meant the former Berlin colleague visited the Kempers twice in Brazil. In turn, Kemper ignored the infighting back home that in the showdown between Müller-Braunschweig and Schultz-Hencke created two societies in Berlin, an officially analytic one (the DPV) and the other older one (the DPG) that was redefined by the split as Neo, eclectic, or Greater-Psychoanalytic, in any event a proper heir not of psychoanalysis as such but of its German history.

The happy medium of the transmission that was still possible in the first years right after the war was psychotherapy. Kemper gave the update with destiny in a monograph closer to the time of this transmission than his 1973 retrospective: *Die Seelenheilkunde in unserer Zeit. Ihre Entwicklung, ihr Stand, ihr Anspruch* (Psychotherapy in Our Time. Its Development, Its Standing, Its Aspiration).[7] *Seelenheilkunde*, "doctrine of soul healing," is an all-German word that shows its date mark. A year later for an overview of this matter, specifically in the setting of Berlin, he uses in the title the international word *Psychotherapie*. Kemper commenced composing *Die Seelenheilkunde in unserer Zeit* toward the end of the war (and thus during the span of time following Rittmeister's execution). It was completed, published in and adjusted to the postwar period. But "our time" is continuous with the recent past.

> In the final phase of this terrible war during the battle of Berlin the "Institute for Psychological Research and Psychotherapy" burned down to its foundations in the last days of April 1945 together with all its contents including all the results of years of work. Thus, in just a few hours what had been built up laboriously over decades was destroyed. The germ cell of the institute was the training institute, which together with the clinic was originally set up by the psychoanalytic society in 1920, but which after 1933 during political coordination came to be integrated as supporting framework for the institute mentioned above. Through the amalgamation of all the depth-psychological perspectives the institute became the central collecting point of psychotherapy… With its destruction a fateful concluding line was drawn beneath a development, which in the final years increasingly filled the thoughtful with concern about its hyper-occupied character, which tended to be expansive and intent on efficiency, as conditioned by the pressures of the war years – not to mention the political tendencies reflected therein. This critical standpoint should not, however, cause us to overlook that during this same period despite it all, behind the façade as it were, silently, an inner development transpired, the historical necessity of which was given in the constellation at that time of the still so young scientific field of psychotherapy. This work of development was carried by a numerically small circle and had to be pursued largely hidden from the officially ruling tendencies of the period. The fruitful results of this development are already evident to the informed. They will in the time that lies before us be proved for the first time in their complete range and consequence. Now that the hermetic enclosure has begun to open regarding the research that was being pursued all this time outside Germany, it gives special satisfaction and justification that in the meantime in the rest of the world essentially the same developmental momentum has everywhere begun to assert itself. (7–8)[8]

Kemper retraces through this internal development the analytic reclaiming of the breakaway movements associated with Adler and Jung not in the mode of reunion but to form a more perfect foundation for modern psychotherapy. The return of the split-off perspectives of Adler and Jung introduced analytic psychotherapy or depth psychology by opening the analytic field to a more complete range of therapeutic techniques. Depth psychology – already the eclectic version of original psychoanalysis via Adler and Jung – serves as the control, as Kemper puts it, governing the application of the therapeutic method selected from among the complete range of techniques available in the mental health field as most compatible with a given case to be treated. Kemper rescues an inner development of psychotherapy (what Rittmeister termed a new humanism) from the doomed central Nazi German institute permeated by the malaise that Rittmeister assigned to his own stuck place in life as in his work: over-expansive formulation at the expense of detail.

In the 1947 preface to *Bettnässer-Leiden (Enuresis). Zur Entstehung, Vorbeugung und Behandlung kindlicher Fehlentwicklungen* (Bedwetting Afflictions [Enuresis]. On Etiology, Prevention, and Treatment of Aberrant Developments in Childhood),[9] Kemper extols the teamwork with Schultz-Hencke and the latter's students as making this study possible. In the 1975 preface to the new edition, he explains that the foundation of the study is Freud. But he identifies himself as a second-generation Freudian – together with Anna Freud, Melanie Klein, René Spitz and D.W. Winnicott – also to the extent, he says, that he shifted his research in the direction of the mother-and-infant dyad.

A sort of cleansing (or as Schreber would say, testing) relationship to the milieu of therapeutic eclecticism that Schultz-Hencke owned in postwar Berlin seems to emerge in the relay of prefaces. In a 1949 preface, written and signed in Rio de Janeiro, and appended to his book *Die funktionalen Sexualstörungen* (Functional Sexual Disturbances), Kemper admits that the study was first written as assigned in 1943. It was to be his contribution to a collection of essays on functional disturbances of the different organ systems. But upon its completion, the collection, since deemed not (or no longer) important for the war effort, was not published. The only changes he introduced were to make his work independent of its initial role as part of that total effort.

The 1972 preface to the new edition was written in Berlin. Back to the future: for this edition he rewrote or replaced certain dated formulations that were comprehensible only to those well-versed in Berlin's eclectic therapy scene during the Third Reich as well as in the immediate postwar period. J.H. Schultz, one of the few Göring Institute members whose work survived the Nazi era intact and well-received, gives a positive blurb on the cover.

Three decades ago, when he composed this work "from the vantage point of the director of a Berlin psychotherapy clinic that was analytically oriented" (the position he assumed in 1943), it opened new ground. Of course, there was around the world related research activity in this area but most of it was unavailable to Kemper at the time. The reasons for this restriction are given parenthetically: "(Third Reich, war)."

What he added just the same to this unknown community of research was the open communication he initiated between gynecology and psychotherapy. He started on this path with his 1942 publication *Die Störungen der Liebesfähigkeit beim Weibe* (The Disturbances of the Capacity for Love in the Female). But the times they are in the meantime changing. Kemper refers to a "sex wave" in popular culture and a matching upsurge of soft-porn studies of sexual problems. This spread of sexological understanding and application has not, however, led to a drop but in fact there's been a rise in the incidence of disturbances. The study reflects the onset of psychodynamic treatment of these disorders. Though for reasons of his own he practices now only pure psychoanalysis, Kemper considers publication of this work justified, not only because it documents the beginnings of the now established psychosomatic approach but also on account of the detailed case presentations that include concrete background conditions of these disturbances, which are not largely known.

The study also documents the links and limits of analytically oriented "small psychotherapy" (to borrow again from the lexicon of the Göring Institute). For the wide-ranging application of the newly emerging discipline of social psychology (which Kemper thinks could be more accurately identified as "psycho-social prophylaxis and theory") short-term psychotherapy is once again of great import. But it isn't only the continuity shot of innovations at the Göring Institute that Kemper is projecting. The eclectic therapeutic approach was altered in adaptation to the postwar period by the inclusion or even foregrounding of psychoanalytic group therapy.

Kemper's memoir of his encounter with the otherness of Brazil belabors the Freudian purchase on the German-Romantic motif of the *Doppelgänger*: "Fleeting, almost arbitrary searchlights illuminating a mentality that appeared to us at first very alien, suddenly unmistakably showed us our own image in the mirror of the other."[10] He found himself in a country that the arrival of "plane, telegraph, film, radio, TV and the like" had only recently "shocked" out of the long isolation obtaining since its discovery and colonization in the sixteenth century (5). "The Brazilian lives therefore in a tumultuous condition of preliminarity between becoming and expiring" (5).

> Only by venturing an empathic (*teilhabenden*) identification was I able to immerse myself in what was foreign and grasp it emotionally from within. Only then could I evaluate after the fact and from a reinstated remove that which I had fully lived through as experiences and arrange them according to the connections known to me. – Repeated implementation of resonant identification and psychic confrontation in such constant alternation is also how in my psychotherapeutic work I comprehend what is transpiring in my counterpart, the patient. (4)

What socked him in the eye so he could see better was the force of irrationality for good and evil "in our own past" (4). When he argues that in the setting of Evangelist radio programs the fighting words of the believers, "Jesús está presente!!!," summoning and realizing a magical world that alone is authentic and true, he is reminded of the German masses shouting "Heil Hitler!" not so very long ago (18). Kemper came to pursue the group dynamic that's the silver lining in mass behavior as the best format for psychotherapy in Brazil or in Germany.

Interest in analytic group therapy was something Kemper and his training analysand Cabernite had in common. But Kemper first engaged in group therapy, on improvisational basis, at the postwar Berlin psychotherapeutic clinic he founded and governed together with Schultz-Hencke. According to his 1947 survey of *Seelenheilkunde*, he sought to bind the postwar clinic (and by implication the Göring Institute) via an inner development back to the institute Eitingon founded in 1920. Kemper came to view the deepening of his earlier pragmatic contact with group work as the destinal legacy of his 1948 move to South America where several analysts were actively seeking compatibility with the group format. While on this map, Kemper secured for German translation and publication a Spanish language collection of essays on analytic group therapy edited by the Argentine analysts Leon Grinberg, Marie Langer and Emilio Rodrigué.[11]

In his 1971 preface to the second German edition of *Psychoanalytic Group Therapy*, which (in contrast to the first preface of 1960) reflects the period of his return to Germany, Kemper starts out diagnosing the intervening upsurge in Germany of interest in group therapy evident in countless self-discovery groups. All kinds of group leadership find their match and maker in social upheaval, which in Germany at least, says Kemper, is specifically tied to the gap in generation of ideals. Institutions of higher learning have been undermined or, as Kemper also puts it, secularized by the declining course of a world order that lost all credibility during two world wars. The media, Kemper notes, have spread even to the most isolated village the news of the horrors perpetrated by the old order. Members of this order in turn charge ingratitude and foreground the countertestimony of all their well-meant efforts like the economic miracle. What's more, the uncontrollable conditions of the recent past only implicate a collective evil that lets them individually off the hook. The result is a rebellion of youth against an older generation that cannot recognize any cause for it in the setting of economic, technical and scientific progress.

There are two types of protest. The first involves withdrawal from reality into a fantasy realm, which in its collective momentum alone differs from individual delusion. The second and active variant terroristically targets every authority without respect for property or individual life. Whether item one or item two, the German setting illustrates for Kemper a metapsychological fact: groups border on psychosis. According to Kemper, the analytic approach acknowledges what every encounter with group dynamics involves, namely, just as in the treatment of psychosis, inevitable explosive detonations of forces otherwise bound up in symptoms and related modes of inhibition. The task is to bind these forces anew within a dosage of controlled release.

> We already know from psychoanalytic work with individual patients what powerful drive forces can be thereby released. In their explosive power they have been compared, not inappropriately, to the release of atomic energy. Certain mass phenomena of recent times provided all of us with shattering proofs of the unsuspected massive impact of forces slumbering potentially in collectives – and which can be released for good or bad.

Special controls are needed when working with these atomic or group energies. Otherwise, such harmful results follow, Kemper advises, as "fateful short circuit reactions (acting outs) in professional or private life, the breaking out of neurotic or psychosomatic symptoms, the becoming manifest of a psychosis, all the way to so-called unexplained suicides." To harness the energies spread out before him Kemper reassigns to the analytic group its, as he says, little known special task. At the same time, he flashes back to the Göring Institute, where the distinction was drawn and observed between long-term individual analytic psychotherapy, referred to, by analogy with surgery, as "big psychotherapy" and so-called small psychotherapy, which included any number of short-term therapies.

> As is well known, the observations and experiences made in big psychoanalytic individual therapy contributed after the fact to the understanding of what transpires in so-called small psychotherapy, in which by and large psychotherapeutic methods of the pre-analytic era are tried out, and what element therein can be addressed as the effective force or agent. Only in this way could the possibilities and the limits of every one of these psychotherapeutic approaches be demarcated and trustworthy statements made, and standards upheld regarding selection and mode of application of the optimal psychotherapeutic approach indicated for each individual case. Thus psychoanalysis, originally simply a method of treatment, became, after the fact, to borrow for the purpose of illumination a comparison from technology, a test site or experimental laboratory for related methods of treatment; and not with the aim of secretly retooling them as analytic methods, but rather to make generally available already existing specialized insights and experiences.

In a footnote dropped in 1959 for the German edition, the co-authors from Argentina note that colleague Kemper implemented didactic group analysis as a required part of the training of candidates at the analytic institute he founded and presided over in Rio de Janeiro.

In the preface to his 1964 study *Der Traum und seine Be-Deutung* (Dream and Its Significance/Interpretation) Kemper signs in as "orthodox psychoanalyst." It is an identification that the history of his involvement in emplacing Freud's science within an environment of eclectic psychotherapy would seem to contradict. And yet, even though its separateness or autonomy could never really be defined or located, psychoanalysis still played a leading role in all his efforts to secure the testing and selection of therapeutic techniques for the best possible fit between a client's affliction and the format and method of psychotherapeutic treatment. And when he left for Brazil, he left behind the German history of psychoanalysis and joined instead international psychoanalysis, the new orthodoxy.

Notes

1 Schultz-Hencke put out his shingle postwar as Neo analyst in a context shared with colleague Karen Horney. Like Heinz Hartmann and Wilhelm Reich, he underwent his didactic analysis with Sándor Radó, who in the postwar era also came to count as Neo analyst.

2 Werner Kemper, "Werner Kemper," *Psychotherapie in Selbstdarstellungen*, ed. Ludwig J. Pongratz (Bern: Verlag Hans Huber, 1973), 277. The subsequent page references are given in the text.

3 One platform of the dissidents during the psychoanalytic controversy in Rio de Janeiro in the 1980s was the eradication of the distinction between psychoanalyst and didactic psychoanalyst, the distinction that brought Kemper to Brazil.
4 Bräutigam, *John Rittmeister*, 31.
5 See *"Hier geht das Leben...,"* ed. Karen Brecht et al., 170, 172. The stipend and ticket had already been given him but no explanation when the trip was suddenly prohibited. He was arrested in September.
6 Werner W. Kemper, *Archaische Kräfte im Schmelztiegel Brasilien* (Archaic Forces in Melting Pot Brazil) (Bremen: Angelsachsen-Verlag, 1965), 3.
7 *Die Seelenheilkunde in unserer Zeit. Ihre Entwicklung, ihr Stand, ihr Anspruch* (Stuttgart: Klett Verlag, 1947). Page references are given in the text.
8 In *Die Reinigung der Psychoanalyse*, 57–58, Lockot refers to a document that a member of the institute, Cäcilie Olten, entrusted to Schultz-Hencke regarding the details of the day the Göring Institute burned to the ground. Indeed, it was during the Soviet conquest of Berlin. But this was when Matthias Göring was captured, his staff failing or refusing to bury the insignia of his National Socialist affiliation. A sniper shot at the Soviet soldiers, and they rounded everyone else up, placed them in the cellar and set the building on fire. But there was a bombing induced opening in the cellar wall, and the institute staff and members escaped, Erna Göring leading the way, convinced that they were still being aided by the SS. Kemper's description of the destruction of the institute in 1973 lumps the event together with last major air raids. In 1947 he describes it differently. The institute may have been largely destroyed before the Soviet soldiers put a match to it. Even the Adlon Hotel, although bombed to an unrecognizable fragment of its former street view, was still used before it too was demolished. That Lockot attempts to make of these variants a demo of Kemper's ambivalence is a good example of the detective work his case has attracted.
9 Werner W. Kemper, *Bettnässer-Leiden (Enuresis). Zur Entstehung, Vorbeugung und Behandlung kindlicher Fehlentwicklungen* (Munich and Basel: Ernst Reinhardt Verlag, 1978).
10 Werner W. Kemper, *Archaische Kräfte im Schmelztiegel Brasilien* (Bremen: Angelsachsen-Verlag, 1965), 18. The subsequent page references are given in the text.
11 *Psychoanalytische Gruppentherapie. Praxis und theoretische Grundlage*, trans. A. Freund and G. Krichhauff (Munich: Kindler Verlag, 1972). Kemper edited and introduced the German edition. Page references to the introduction are given in the text.

Chapter 8

Schweigen and Giving Them the Slips

In three issues from the early run of *PSYCHE*, the journal that Alexander Mitscherlich founded in 1947 together with Hans Kunz and Felix Schottlaender, Werner Kemper published work that reached back into his recent past at the Göring Institute in Nazi Berlin. Mitscherlich was putting out his shingle in the role of Freud's champion, facilitating the alleged return of psychoanalysis. But Mitscherlich came from psychosomatic medicine and trained as an analyst only after all his opening seasons of pretending to be an international analyst. *PSYCHE* stepped in where Carl Müller-Braunschweig's postwar journal, *Zeitschrift für Psychoanalyse* (Journal for Psychoanalysis), left off after two issues. We will be looking long and hard at the vintage Kemper articles that Müller-Braunschweig published and introduced as historical documents awaiting integration within postwar German psychoanalysis.

Kemper gives a historical introduction to his first *PSYCHE* publication in 1948. But in the longer run, it seems, Mitscherlich and co. just didn't want to go there and historicize a past that for better or worse didn't comply with their agenda of discontinuity and return. We begin with the second article, also published in 1948, which Kemper didn't contextualize, and so we don't know when or how it was rehearsed, unlike the first article, which Kemper notes was a lecture he presented four years earlier at the Göring Institute.

Given that two generations of training analysts and analysands had allegedly run aground in the silence Kemper kept in Rio about his time in Nazi Berlin, his critics saw the article as scandalously giving how-to instruction in adjusting to an untenable situation.[1] While Besserman Vianna and Major's reading of the transference and transfer between Nazi Berlin and Rio de Janeiro does hold, it doesn't transmit Kemper's culpability. However, it's one thing to judge on paper that the German analysts did try to maintain Freud's science. It's something else again to act on it and send one of those German analysts to a foreign land to act as founding father of a new chapter in the history of psychoanalysis. What does surface in the third generation, as manifest in the discourse of Amilcar Lobo, is a linguistic blend of brutal and precious affirmations of the truth and nothingness of thriving in surviving.

The less tendentious charge is that Kemper was an opportunist and impostor. One exhibit for the prosecution is this brief text on the *Schweigen* or keeping silent

DOI: 10.4324/9781003797708-11

that patients at times manifest. The essay shows a readiness to adapt the talking cure, however subtly and carefully, to the realities of political pressures. The cone of confidentiality that protects free association in psychoanalysis becomes a loop of suspicion in the paranoid milieu of treating patients under conditions of totalitarianism. So, in lieu of the rule of free association, Kemper stipulated that his patients must state in the session whenever they felt constrained to maintain silence. The essay can also be enlisted for the defense. Kemper was proud of his brief article and saw to it that it was translated into Portuguese. Judged by Rickman and Jones uncontaminated by the National Socialist ideology that he had navigated for the duration, Kemper was entitled to his minority report that it was by containing the impingement of the patient keeping silent in session that the work of analysis could continue.[2]

"Der Patient schweigt" (The Patient Keeps Silent) opens in the style of "The Uncanny" with a philological turn to and through the *Muttersprache*, in which we can find lost connections that resonate with the history of words.[3] At the same time it's like a technical paper that revises or supplements the basic rule of speaking and associating freely in session. By looking at all the meanings of silence and silencing indwelling the history and the unconscious of words, Kemper makes a clearing for therapeutic adjustments to a setting too paranoid and violent for integrating a trustworthy and working sense of confidentiality.

Not all speaking undoes silence and secrecy. Talking like a waterfall (*Redeflut*) is the best way to hide something (508). There are also those with a lazy mouth (*die Mundfaulen*) and others who are sparse of words (*die Wortkargen*). Every speaking that expresses and externalizes is a *Hergeben*, a giving away, a loss of substance. Neither keeping nor receiving, the situation of letting go is so difficult for the neurotic (509). Whether or not talkative, neurotically ill people are steeped in the unconscious of language; they experience in an exchange of words an ancillary amplification of the "symbolic-magical cathexis of word and speech act" (505), which can get in the way of communication. Instead, spoken language acquires a symbolic function and can conjure, curse or silence. The witch was believed to be a cattle whisperer, whose bespeaking, however, could also make the animals sick. The fairy-tale motif of the power of speech swabs over into expressions like talking to death, biting one's tongue, or the evil tongue of defamation (*üble Nachrede*) (517).

A weapon in session, keeping silent is the negative to the positive of saying whatever is on your mind, the fundamental law of Freudian analysis. Silence can magically shake the infantile sense of the analyst's omnipotence and test his omniscience (512). This reaches back to the child's early experience that lying skips the purview of the parents. Kemper sketches a typology of *Schweigen* to guide work with clients across the obstacle course of secrecy. Helpless silence reflects disappointment in the therapist and leads to a feeling of loss of contact (513). Evasive silence tries to deal with the loss of contact (514). The silence of the analyst is golden but the patient who keeps silent casts in copper and tin difficulties and disturbances in making and maintaining the connection (510–511). Analysts forget that the demand to tell all in session goes against nature just like certain moments in a gynecological exam. The demand on the patient is to spell and spill it all out, including impulses, wishes, fantasies, even bodily sensations, and perceptions (507).

You can kill a topic by talking it to death (*tot-reden*) or by keeping silent. Among the topics killed in session are not only those sexually themed but even more so all that orbits anality, including money and property. That there are "official secrets" (*Dienstgeheimnisse)* as well is a reference to the time and place of the text's composition (506). To protect a third party, a patient keeps quiet about his complicit knowledge of criminal matters, especially if the therapist knows the third person in question. Before launching the quest for the meaning of what was silenced, the keeping silent itself must be addressed and understood (521). Keeping silent like not dreaming, coming late to the session and forgetting a whole session resists the work of the analysis. (He refers to Wilhelm Reich as an astute reader of negative transferences.)

In a situation of multiple layers of silence and secrecy, it is important that the patient say when he is keeping something back – like "no comment." More important in a police state setting is that the moment of keeping silent in session be admitted and known. Having gone this far, Kemper is charmed by the prospect of writing a companion piece titled "Der Therapeut schweigt" (518), which would complete the investigation of the therapeutic aspects of keeping silent in the transference.

This is a good place to underscore that Matthias Göring could not be confided in by colleagues at the institute who were treating patients whose speech acts and related activities might be construed as treasonous. Ludger Hermanns documents this condition of not being able to discuss case material openly in group, that is, not being able to share anything that could be considered of political significance. It wasn't possible to trust the non-analysts at the institute who were more likely to sacrifice therapeutic discretion to the greater cause. You had to present your case to Göring but if there was anything among the details of the case that smacked of political betrayal (like the theft of weapons by a 14-year-old under treatment at the institute for antisocial tendencies) then you could be sure that "Papa" (his moniker among the clinicians) would break confidentiality. The teen being treated by Marianne Stark was already charged in a court case and the evidence Göring gleaned from her discussion of the case and duly reported meant that only with the greatest effort could he be saved from the euthanasia meted out for such a serious crime.[4] Göring's eagerness to prosecute patients even for defeatism, Ludger Hermanns concludes, necessarily hindered the "productivity" of the psychoanalysts in their practice. It was all along the globally anticipated condition of always possible governmental constraint that was the reason Freud enjoined analysts to refrain from making their politics public.

Under the Brazilian military dictatorship that took over in 1964, to come full circle, analysis flourished to a degree unparalleled in the modern history of the country. Does political oppression make the safeguarding of confidentiality a less ambiguous enterprise and increase the productivity in session? Hermanns considers the prohibition of the professional analytic language and its inseparable metapsychology and the consequent imposition of a camouflage discourse, in which the designations of the concepts known to the analysts had to be cumbersomely rewritten, another blocker of analytic productivity.[5] This applies to the publications as well as to the eclectic meetings with the therapists from other schools (many of whom were Nazis) but not to the in-group discussions among the analysts when they were on their own. Hermanns's inspired suggestion that those young analysts who were raised and trained under the aegis of the "slave language" suffered a loss of substance in the content of their understanding and practice[6] says more about the next generation of West German psychoanalysts who were educated by those analysts so adept at adopting camouflage selves and discourses that they just couldn't stop after the war.

The third and shortest article, "Mehrzeitige Fehlhandlungen" (Lapses at Multiple Times), which appeared in *PSYCHE* in 1949, already gave Kemper's address as Rio de Janeiro. In the contemporary setting Kemper recognized that the research and technical interest in slips of the tongue and other lapses had subsided and, if anything, awakened a kind of friendly-sad memory of the good old days.[7] "More convincing and effortless than the study of dreams, certainly than the study of neurotic symptomatology, was the uncovering of the hidden meanings of apparently senseless and random lapses, which also led outsiders to a first understanding of certain depth-psychological connections" (77). But today's tendency is a mistake: especially at the start of an analysis a lapsus can signal the inner disposition of the patient and contribute to working on the transference.

He gives his case example of a multiple lapsus happening at different times, which dates back 15 years, and belongs to the opening years of the Third Reich (78). The patient was a 35-year-old artist, her personality structure was infantile-oral, and her slow-going treatment was, of late, belaboring the theme of money. She enjoins him to accept his therapeutic work as a calling, as his being called, like her own vocation as artist, without complying with or passing along "dirty" financial transactional demands. She for one would never take money for what she's called to do, nor has she ever done anything just for the money (79). What's not directly addressed is that she pays Kemper for a Jewish treatment and through all this talk of dirty money in the setting of state anti-Semitism the patient is calling – in synch or swim with the hate that's in the air – for a fantastic breaching of a technical rule that is as basic as the injunction to speak openly and freely.

That afternoon she helps a woman in her building who's ill by going to make a payment of 120 Reichsmark on her behalf. When it's time to pay, she's short 20 Reichsmark. She's perfectly capable of losing money without a trace and so she borrows the missing amount from her sister to make the payment. But the episode weighs on her and when her mother and sister notice and ask her what's wrong she relates the mishap. Her sister tells the woman whom the patient was helping what happened and when she double checks, presto, she finds the money she inadvertently never gave her emissary. The patient is delighted to find in this incident further proof that money need be for her neither object nor subject and looks forward to rubbing Kemper's nose in it.

Next day she awaits change from the 20 Reichsmark bill she presented in payment and the shopkeeper says she hasn't paid him yet. Tensions rise (back home she curses him a dirty moneygrubber) but since she is a regular customer he goes along with her version of events. Why does this sort of thing always happen to her! Then on the following day in session, she relates both episodes to Kemper. Excited, upset, starting to cry, she yanks from her purse the hanky that lets fly the missing Reichsmark bill. The patient is struck, stunned, but gets it (80). What the interpretation of her dreams and the analysis of her behavior couldn't achieve, this multiple lapsus brought about instantly, opening the impasse between her noble indifference to money and a grandiosity that denies that there will be bills to pay. Upon the bursting of the dam (80) their work together begins to flow unto a happy ending in therapeutic resolution.

Notes

1 See Hans Füchner on "Der Fall Werner Kemper." Already by shoring up the organization in Berlin after the expulsion of the Jewish colleagues, the psychoanalysts who stayed and continued to work at the institute, including Kemper, had made an untenable adjustment. That said, however, Füchner shows that all the other sensational charges don't apply to Kemper. He considers a highly critical publication by a certain Mattos in Brazil that focuses on Kemper's article on the patient keeping silent. Füchner can blame the sloppy translation at one point: what Kemper carefully designates as his hybrid psychoanalytic-psychotherapeutic approach is given in Portuguese as a purely psychoanalytic one. But for the most part the Mattos monograph reflects ill will and the reflex response of closing ranks. The overriding local-to-global interpretation of the torture scandal in Rio as the consequence of Kemper's personal history, traits and behavior must be rejected outright.

2 Can the patient forced by the reality of the political situation to keep silent in session silence history? Bernard A. Kamm didn't stay around to find out. The only gentile analyst to join his Jewish colleagues in exile in 1935 responded in 1980 to Regine Lockot's dissertation-research inquiries, writing that the analysis of neurosis isn't possible if the environment in which the sessions are held is as restrictive or more so than the original threatening home situation. The analyst would be deceiving and endangering his patient and himself if he behaved as though everything in and around the session can be freely thought through and expressed. "Both analyst and analysand must remain conscious of the fact that nothing can remain secret in such an environment dominated by paranoia and that at any point denunciation can follow upon suspicion alone." Who can prove in such an inimical situation that thoughts don't lead to acts? See Christine Trollope, trans., *"Here Life Goes on in a Most Peculiar Way..." Psychoanalysis Before and After 1933* (Hamburg: Kellner Verlag, 1992), 164.

3 Werner Kemper, "Der Patient schweigt," *PSYCHE*, 1, 4 (May 1948), 503–522; here 503. The subsequent page references are given in the text.

4 Ludger M. Hermanns, "Bedingungen und Grenzen wissenschaftlicher Produktivität bei Psychoanalytikern in Deutschland 1933 bis 1945 – mit einem exemplarischen Versuch über Alexander Mette und sein Novalis-Projekt," *Jahrbuch der Psychoanalyse*, 25 (1989), 28–54; here: 29.

5 Hermanns, "Bedingungen und Grenzen," 30.

6 Hermanns, "Bedingungen und Grenzen," 30.

7 Werner Kemper, "Mehrzeitige Fehlhandlungen," *PSYCHE*, 3, 1 (1949), 77–80; here: 77.

Chapter 9

Hard on the Trail of the Missing

The first *PSYCHE* article by Kemper, his 1948 "Verdrängte Vitalität – Zur Symptomatik des Priapismus" (Repressed Vitality – On the Symptomatology of Priapism), dates back to 1944 when he presented it to his *Arbeitskreis* or working group at the Göring Institute.[1] What the circumstances of the air war necessitated in the short term, namely, the abbreviation or condensation of the treatment, compromises in the long term his use of this case as an instance of analytic work: the gold of the analytic stance was interpenetrated by the copper of suggestion (412).

At the time Kemper started taking down his patient's history, the events of the war had one year earlier brought about the evacuation of the patient's home life to the countryside, while he remained with his day job in the city. His respite from the workplace was reduced to weekend visits every two or four weeks (414). For Kemper, the patient's presenting problem is the impasse he can't integrate or get around between asceticism and masturbation. The patient presents the symptom of his priapism.

During adolescence he suffered from a developing phimosis. In a dream he recalls from his student days (he wanted to become a pastor but then switched from the preaching to the teaching profession) he is playing the organ with both hands but not a tone is to be heard (no doubt, Kemper surmises, because the bellows didn't blow, a message, Kemper notes to himself, from the gastrointestinal underworld) (417).

When the patient was 14 the developing phimosis stimulated and prompted masturbation. By age 19 his condition had worsened and the urge to masturbate was a dangerous temptation (415). Two years before his marriage, his cousin, a surgeon, removed the phimosis leaving only a limited "distortion" (*Entstellung*), which amounts, in other words, to the discrete marking of circumcision (414).

The night before the second session he has his first wet dream in almost two years: A radiant light like a gloriole outlines his wife's figure against her night clothes and she's looking good like a magnificent sculpture should (418). He lies awake in the afterglow and goo enjoying fantasy images that are erotic rather than sexual, involving an "ecstatically heightened experience of the harmony of the world" (419). Kemper observes that in producing a halo effect the light show suggested a religious experience, but that it also made the wife's garment see-through.

DOI: 10.4324/9781003797708-12

But since in his dream the patient is lying on his back in his mother's bed, he has not yet assumed the paternal position of independent masculinity.

It's the third session and the patient is being evasive. Kemper asks for any dreams. Yes, he had a dream in which he was at the dentist's office waiting to have his tooth pulled. Although he knows better, the fear of the pain gets the upper hand, and he keeps his mouth shut. Does he or doesn't he want his truth pulled? What the patient calls his *Vitalschicht* (stratum of vitality) and Kemper the biological order relates to his physical well-being like the rhythm to the beat. Switching the analogizing to the medium of projection, Kemper concludes: "The lively film that's playing is composed out of a sum of static individual images, and yet their summation doesn't add up to the specifics of a moving 'living' film" (420–421). The biological order follows laws, and it is as much a sin to break them, Kemper suggests, as is, for the patient, transgressing against the tenets of his Christian faith (421).

Kemper must cancel the next session because his office took a direct hit in the last air raid (421). A few days later Kemper learns in a letter that his patient has been sleeping the night through and although upon awakening he has the wood it's not a symptom. He even napped a few times without waking up with an erection. Unhappily his deep sleep hasn't yielded dreams he can remember. One brief exception is the serial dream that continues to pop up even during this dry spell. It encompasses the phrase passing through his sleeping head: "mother is dead." The difference is that in the past he would be tortured by the thought upon awakening. Not so now. It leaves him indifferent. Does that mean the maternal influence is dissipating? End of letter.

He spent time with his wife since writing the letter and in the fourth session he relates an instance of premature ejaculation but then, when they tried again, the copulation was successful. Afterwards in bed he suffered the priapism, but it wasn't as painful as usual. He snatched the shred of a dream that was erotically charged. But the plump dream girl, says the patient, isn't at all his type in waking reality. Kemper reminds him that the earlier illuminated wet dream had given his super slender wife curves (422). When asked for associations with the full-size girl he recalls a housekeeper he admired when he was 11 and then withdraws behind a smile. Kemper persists. The patient admits that he was thinking of a vital colleague with whom he's been working closely for two years now. Although he always valued her as a colleague, only recently has he started to find her fascinating despite (Kemper adds an exclamation point) her curvaceousness. The word for "in spite of," *trotz*, also means, when capitalized, "defiance." Twice recently he arranged to meet with her to go for a stroll.

The night before there was a dream to remember, he almost forgot. He was in his hometown at a railroad underpass. Various colleagues joined him, bringing along food to eat. They chose the important transportation intersection as the best spot for their meeting. But something was still lacking to make it all right. What are his associations with the railway intersection? In childhood he was thrilled to watch from above the arrival and departure of trains and got especially excited when the heavily laden freight train's locomotive puff puffed along and engulfed him in its smoke cloud (423). His technical and mathematical interests, Kemper nods as we nod off, must come from this childhood pastime and pleasure. But doesn't the two-level intersection convey the import of uniting his vital and spiritual aspects? He described three levels, Kemper points out, and the patient agrees that there are three aspects that await integration.

In session number five he rejects Kemper's approach from the vantage of his own *Weltanschauung* as too materialistic (423–424). Kemper ignores the reproach and asks him about any dreams. Yes, he was in a bathtub that was threatening to overflow, and he started a counterwave movement to hold the water in check, but the water's surging (*Wogen*) proved ever stronger. Then he's on the surface of a vast ocean and the waves (*Wogen*) are now house-high (424). In his associations it becomes clear that it's less a dread of drowning that's the special feature of the horror dream and more the uncanny sensation of being grabbed and dragged down by something overpowering. Before the night dream he had been on a walk with his colleague, felt moved by her uninhibited friendliness and sensed that his usual stiff (*steif*) self was loosening up. And then she kissed him. They're both married. A second dream that same night. Caught in a downpour he finds safety in the living room of his parents and listens to the rushing sounds (*Rauschen*) of the rain pounding outside. That same night there was a third dream, too, and it was about dreaming (425). He says he's going to dictate his dreams to his colleague so she can type them up for Dr. Kemper. But then he realizes that his comely colleague might then know too much about him and he drops the idea of her recording service.

Everything that happens in this case study is inflected and staggered by keeping silent. We can appreciate how the article on *Schweigen*, which is devoid of case examples, amounts to Kemper's metapsychological reckoning with the fundamental changes the Nazi state introduced into the working relationship to the unconscious.

In the sixth session the patient relates a dream in which he visited his brother who was in the hospital waiting to be vaccinated. The dreamer decides he can do it and applies the needle to the vaccine container, turning the contents blue and brown. When the nurse (*Schwester*) arrives and announces that the doctor is on his way, he tells her what happened, that his brother shouldn't be prosecuted for the contamination of the vaccine. She laughs and says Dr. Y. (who is also the patient's boss) knows everything and will put everyone in the proper place (426). During free association, it emerges that Dr. Y. resembles Kemper.

Kemper says the patient's brother, his own flesh and blood, is his "alter ego," which in German, allow me to add in silent partnership, is also his "old" ego. The patient doesn't want to entrust his old ego's treatment to the doctor, Kemper's lookalike. By administering the inoculation and controlling the dosage he feels he won't be subjected to the house-high waves rolling in from the unknown. The patient responds to the interpretation with a laughing attack that rhythmically increases, convulsively finding release. This is not at all like the patient and signals unconscious confirmation.

When the patient leaves, Kemper notes a new awkwardness in their contact (427). Kemper drops inside a footnote that the largish inoculating device containing fluid colored blue and brown hangs between his own legs and the patient wants to and doesn't want to submit passively to its potency (427 n1).

Prior to session number seven the patient spent a few vacation days with his wife and a dream stayed with him. His wife and daughter point out to him the rabbits hopping happily in the distance. But he next recognizes two wild boars, which leap into the river and swim to shore. The vista vanishes. A donkey stands before him making odd movements of lust and thrust, even though the female animal is nearby. It puzzles the dreamer but then on closer inspection he sees that the donkey's male organ is tightly bound in cloth, whereupon he awoke with a powerful erection but not yet at the point of ejaculation (428). He feels disgust and indignation at the sadistic treatment of the creature being kept from having a proper erection and sexual release.

The patient volunteers that he is the donkey and that a fold in the bed sheet had wrapped up his penis and triggered the dream. Kemper ignores the daily residue and says that the remote vista in his dream denotes the past of childhood wherein the rabbits, well known to be fecund and voracious, innocently play. What comes closer with the wild boars is the opening era of teenage masturbation. The bound donkey represents the developmental phase the patient now occupies. Even though he opened the discussion by identifying with the donkey, he takes exception to his analyst's closing flourish. But then he reports that his friendship with the other woman is becoming intense and tense: she "devours him too much" and he cherishes his independence – especially at his place of work. Judging by his embarrassment Kemper says outright that the patient is keeping something back.

It was in the sixth session that he didn't tell the analyst that when his female colleague visited him in his room, he was ready for action, for once actively pursuing the object, but because she wasn't feeling well (i.e., was menstruating) nothing came of it. He recalls that in the early years of his marriage he was especially turned on when his wife was having her period. His special excitement, which makes him an active suitor, is a Jewish taboo, a curse on his circumcised penis. Otherwise, he and his wife had sex only when she did the initiating. The nurse or sister, the figure in the dream he brought to the sixth session and who stands in for the female colleague, assures him that the doctor will sort out the primal scene and assign everyone their proper position.

The reflex of convulsive laughter accompanies his admission that he left a dream out of last session's discussion because its reference to an embarrassing incident was too clear. The dreamer is recovering from an operation on his nose, and the nurse says it's not as it should be and wants to summon the professor. When the dreamer-patient argues against it, she takes the cotton out of his nostrils, causing him pain. The professor arrives and determines that all is as it should be. This night dream occurred before the morning dream about the donkey. The patient volunteers that the nose is his penis. Although Kemper knows that the nose knows he asks the patient how he knows this. He cites the idiom that says the size of a man's nose gives away the proportions of his Johannes (his Johnson). His nose-penis is growing, however, like in the Pinocchio lie detector text. What he has been withholding is that the collegial friendship has become intimate. Who knows how long he's been going for walks on the wide side of her buxom body? On the occasion represented in the dream, what started out exciting in their lovemaking was dampened by her wild manipulation of his penis, which caused him pain. He pulled back and didn't climax.

He brings to the eighth session new material for interpreting his donkey identification, which his dream the night before delivered (430). In bed with his wife the special lighting effect returned and gave her curves. He's aroused. She climbs up onto the bed. He lies on his back, and she steps weightlessly onto his face. He grabs her hips but since his penis is caught in his nightshirt he ejaculates before he can enter her. Why in association with the donkey dream had he not remembered that whenever the priapism was so severe that it disturbed his rest, he tried helping himself by loosely wrapping a rough strip of cloth around his flaccid penis?

In his youth the patient was a jock but then desisted to focus on controlling his masturbatory tendencies. This resulted in the loss of his "body feeling" (which the rhythm and beat of his outbursts of laughter repress and represent). His was not a harmoniously loose form but was instead riveted to mechanical rigidity, befitting the self-destructive fight in which he was engaged against the natural vital impulse of a healthy man on behalf of an "ideology that is inimical to instinct and life" (430).

Session nine opens with the patient's observation that his wife, who is currently visiting him, has changed, become more flexible, has loosened up (433). The patient has also been offered a better position but in a town so far away that their sessions can't be continued. Kemper asks the patient if he brought a dream along. Yes. A bear swims in a body of water nearby. Another man has a fright when the bear emerges and grabs his shock of hair, shaking him, and with a laugh pronounces in a human voice: "I just wanted to scare you so you can see better that I'm not a wild animal." The man is flummoxed but the bear is happy and easygoing and trolls along and away.

When the patient expresses the parallel between the bear dream and the other animal dream, Kemper underscores that this time, by contrast, it's an animal suggestive of male potency, not inhibited like the donkey nor regressed and playful like the rabbits (433). Kemper is particularly gratified when his patient, who despite some "personality deformation" around his *Kernneurose* (kernel neurosis, a term coined by his famous colleague at the Göring Institute, J.H. Schultz) was a relatively easy case, brings up in their last session his sense that the held-back urge to urinate and the pressure of gas in the other tract contributed to his priapic symptom (434). The organ playing and the locomotive dreams already communicated this underworld of causation to Kemper, but he withheld commenting on it. Before this breakthrough in the presenting symptom, Kemper listed the further directions in which their work might have gone, arguing that he hadn't foregrounded these aspects because by their schedule alone, punctuated by the air-raids on Berlin, the focus had to be fixed on treating the symptom. When he remarks parenthetically that in all the bedroom dreams the patient is lying on his back like a woman, one is left wondering whether he also never mentioned this to the patient. At the end of the paragraph of Kemper's misgivings that the therapy had to stop here, although in the end the ending of the symptom must be counted a therapeutic success, he drops a footnote to one impacted area in the patient's psyche that they didn't explore: his childhood relationship to his younger brother, who enters the dreams with the animals that come in pairs and are associated with voracious eating. Even in the summary last session Kemper decides "for therapeutic reasons" not to communicate to the patient any of these thoughts around the brother theme (434 n1). The therapist kept silent.

That leaves the god Priapus invoked by the patient's presenting symptom. The son of Dionysus and Aphrodite, he was a fertility deity, a garden gnome bearing a large permanent erection. With it he punish-fucked thieving boys and girls. The donkey was this god's official sacrificial animal. That Priapus enjoyed a second career, already in ancient Greece and Rome, steering merchant vessels clear of misfortune can be aligned with priapism's role in the therapy, allowing Kemper to navigate their work successfully toward improvement of the patient's sex life. The brother gnome and the gastrointestinal underworld could be circumnavigated as well as the Jewish crown that the patient's priapism wore. The patient struggles with his own "idealism" to benefit from the "materialism" of the analyst's "Jewish" ideology. The sessions engorge between the restraining lines the untenable identification with the Jews, berated by the Nazis as big-nosed oversexed priapic gnomes. Lowering the anti, the Jew is the patient's brother.

The brother does show up in the second dream the patient brought along to the last session. The dreamer is newlywed and meets a colleague, who is likewise a recent groom. With their brides in hand, they go to meet his brother and another colleague and their wives for a round of drinks. The wedding ban is issued and denied until the dream is crowded with couples like a group of swingers. Kemper finds it noteworthy that the pleasure outing takes place on a Sunday. Indeed, I would underscore, it's the one detail that makes this a night dream and not a daytime fantasy. His Christian idealism is loosening, making the holy day a fun day. But isn't he also walking in the shadow of the missing Sunday clientele, the Jews?

Note

1 Werner Kemper, "Verdrängte Vitalität – Zur Symptomatik des Priapismus," *PSYCHE*, 1, 3 (1948), 411–435; here: 412. The subsequent page references are given in the text.

Chapter 10

The Transferential Imperative and Homosexuality as Resistance

Käthe Dräger, the psychoanalyst who, secretly a communist, remained discretely in the background during the Nazi years, was, by all accounts, the most level-headed witness to the proceedings in the foreground. She singled out two Kemper articles published postwar in Müller-Braunschweig's *Zeitschrift für Psychoanalyse*: since they were originally presented at the Göring Institute, they document the extent to which psychoanalytic research was still possible under adverse conditions of imposed conformity.[1] It was less the political situation of the Nazi regime and more the institute's imperative of cooperation among the psychotherapies that impinged on the public communication of psychoanalytic work.

On May 10, 1939, Kemper gave a paper at an evening gathering of psychotherapists from all the schools represented at the German Institute of Psychological Research and Psychotherapy, which was published postwar: "Die Übertragung. Ihre diagnostischen und therapeutischen Möglichkeiten" (Transference. Its Diagnositic and Therapeutic Possibilities).[2] Kemper announces that he will be attempting "with emphasis on the genetic-causal viewpoint" to present the transference "independently of theoretical explication" as "matter of fact" (*Tatbestand*) and "empirical experiential property" (*Erfahrungsgut*) which can be "practically tested for its soundness" (99). But to do so we must first advance from the common view of the transference as "servile love dependency" to its real significance as a "normal and ubiquitous psychic phenomenon of a projective nature" (99–100). Transference, he underscores, is not a "desktop speculation" (*Schreibtischspekulation*) but an experiential fact (100).

His first case examples show transference ruining the chance at love. For example, one patient kept falling in love only to fly into a rage after a short time, throwing out the recently beloved, now a "witch." But then he could fall in love with her all over again (102). This switching of sides began to surface in the relationship to Kemper, who knew the history. The patient's mother died when he was four years old. Then an aunt who spoiled him ran the household, followed by a grandmother, another spoiler alert, who was an oddball. Then his father remarried, and the uncontrolled beauty was at best abrupt with the boy. During the developmentally significant span of years in early childhood, then, the patient experienced four very different women in the mother position. This was the model for

DOI: 10.4324/9781003797708-13

the *Durcheinander* – disarrangement, confusion, mix-up – he transferred to his relationships with women, and which also surfaced in the transference relationship to the analyst (102).

"Everything that happens in the doctor–patient relationship can have a transferential character – but doesn't have to, of course" (103). Kemper allows that the doctor–patient relationship is of course a real human relationship. But transference reactions can "flow" into it just the same as into a "riverbed" (*Strombett*) and this "foreign stream" follows certain "laws" (103). The psychoanalyst is trained to read the entirety of the material the patient brings to session, including fantasies and dreams, for the transference content. The analyst knows when the patient is holding back and must draw the patient's attention to this omission. "Only in this way does he not forgo for possible diagnostic therapeutic use the wide-open flow of the transference stream with all its nuances, although one must also take into consideration that the omission itself... can be of transferential significance" (104).

Moving along from what Kemper refers to as his "historical-descriptive representation" in the first part of his paper, which he illustrated with case histories and critical commentaries, he now asks what it is that a patient transfers in the transference. What is transferred is unfinished and unresolved, for example the earliest attempts to master conflicts that were false solutions of a neurotic type (105). The transference conveys both the task itself and the insufficient attempt by the ego to carry it out. But the experience of fantasy can also be transferred. That's why in the transference onto the analyst something announces itself that no longer accords with grown-up thinking and feeling (106). It's a moment that makes the already unreal quality of the transference even more fantastic. The analyst is thus afforded an inside view of the patient as a young child. One of Kemper's patients was coiled up on the couch ready to run away because he saw his analyst as the wolf that had already swallowed his sister (who died in childhood).

Although Kemper continues to treat the transference phenomenon as something that can be controlled, the more cursory or "historical" introduction gives way to the main agenda of his presentation. It's crucial that the analyst "not hinder or warp the transference tendencies in their spontaneous and originary unfolding" (111). The analyst is at once catalyst and representative of reality. The more the analyst can be to the patient a tabula rasa, a blank screen for projections, the more originary the transference phenomena and the more fully they show themselves when projected onto the analyst.

> Beyond this it's important that the developing and soon accruing transference expressions of the patient increase until the optimal maximum is reached for therapeutic fertilization, that is, the analyst must not destroy them in their germination phase by pointing out inadequacies. To achieve this optimum, what's required... is, first, a regular increase, even often an excessive amping up of the transference expressions, which might seem to the outsider outright grotesque... An eruptive breaking out must follow. Only after the evidential experience of such historical forms of relatedness can patients correctly see (*sehen*), that is,

> recognize (*einsehen*) the possibility that it was all inadequate and that their behavior in the current actual transference is of a compulsive nature. A patient is enabled for the first time to break through what was an automatic unconscious operation and open access through constant analytic working-through, allowing the breakthrough to extend to all the significant relations and behaviors outside the analysis. (112)

Patients must enter and become fully aware of the transferential falsification of their world if they are to overcome it therapeutically:

> the patient experiences his behavior as adequate reaction to the world as he sees it, of which the transferential relationship to the analyst represents but a section. And only in the individual case can the analyst gauge how far he must let the patient's transference-falsification go and grow… until the patient experiences the foreign body feeling (*Fremdkörpergefühl*) regarding what he thinks he's doing, which is necessary for the therapeutic fertilization. (112)

In his next case example, Kemper again situates the transference interpretation within the plain text of the patient's history. Her presenting problem is that she doesn't like being a girl and that all her partners dump her: "she has no sense at all how by constantly playing with her partners in a manner that is refined and gruesome she causes each relationship despite another hopeful beginning to fail" (112). The patient asks him to schedule a consultation with her twin brother who's in crisis. Kemper agrees. He doesn't, however, indicate that he knew that by agreeing to see her brother he was triggering what followed. He certainly should have known – and why didn't he refer her brother to a colleague? Right after the consultation with her twin the rapport with the patient changes radically.

Kemper decides not to tell her how ungrounded her suspicions are. He decides to wait it out. She starts showing excessive jealousy toward all his other patients, makes demands on him that are unfulfillable and a cause for endless disappointment. "Parallel to this there is also quiet resentment towards her brother for alleged unkindness toward her" (113). This leads to a break with her twin and to a breakdown. To the patient's surprise, "a totally buried painful world of early childhood comes alive again" (113). It was the time when she played the role of Cinderella in the relationship to her parents and her brother, the long-awaited son and heir. She took flight into her neurotic disposition toward men. Without the byproduct of the negative transference, her questioning of undisturbed and heartfelt relations with her brother, the breakthrough awareness of this buried but therapeutically important world could not have transpired.

The longer the analyst must wait for the unfolding of the negative transference reaction, however, the greater the danger that the patient will justifiably feel that he's being played, even after he comprehends in theory the necessity of the game (114). And yet it is only after the patient lets it all hang out that the analyst can step into his other role as the delegate of reality and dissolve the transference, pointing out the inadequacies and compulsions it carried forward. All this becomes possible only for the analyst who has all along offered a blank screen in which the patient can see it all circling the drain of a vicious circle. Kemper tampers with the word for lived experiencing, *Erleben*, turning it into *Umleben*, to describe the process of integrating the busted foreign body of the transference reaction.

In an aside to his mixed audience Kemper notes that for the analysts or analytic therapists the work on the transference doesn't diminish the other factors in the process of healing, including the import of dream analysis that remains unchanged. Then he addresses the therapists who target behavior: "It becomes clear that also with the therapeutic fertilization of the transference the practicing, readjusting, 'training' moment is equally indispensable" (114). Earlier he included an aside to Pavlov's law of conditioned reflex (107).

He balances these concessions against his orthodox claim that for the work on the transference you need a strictly staged analytic situation, in other words, the couch and no face to face (115). He anticipates the objection that the cold demeanor of the analyst is spooky. But that's not the case, Kemper says, if the analyst offers instead a blank screen. The analyst cannot play act this screen: he must *be* the blank screen. Following his nod to the prejudice against analysis, Kemper continues sorting through the differences between analysis and therapy (at least he places training in quotes): the analyst cannot give directives nor lead the discussion (116). Leave the patient's silence alone; interpret it but don't fill it in. After he says the analyst shouldn't talk about his own life or take examples from his life, he makes a concession to the Adlerian Fritz Künkel, who could still have been in the audience (117).[3] Taking an example from one's own life experience to illustrate a problem a patient is facing in session can be very productive, what Künkel calls the therapeutic We. But it just doesn't apply in the specific situation of the developing transference (117). No matter how careful the analyst is to separate his work from his life, the patient will find out all kinds of things about his analyst. If what the patient makes of what he finds out is interpreted in the session no damage is done. Even in an analysis focused on structural or libidinal problems, which doesn't foreground the transference, any dream that the patient brings to session will bear witness to the transference, which the analyst should be cognizant of even if he doesn't address it in session (119). The analytic work on the transference, Kemper concludes, "achieves the greatest freedom from error (*Fehlerfreiheit*) and amounts to a clear field of testing" (120).

The second Kemper article that appeared in the short-lived journal Müller-Braunschweig founded and edited was particularly recommended by Dräger for its demonstration of what was still possible back then in Nazi Berlin, but she did not identify the article by topic. I was taken by surprise when it was the case study of a patient whose presenting problem was his homosexuality. Like J.H. Schultz, Kemper didn't have to be a specialist in conversion therapy to join in the German mission of understanding homosexuality and making it stand under certain dictates. Like the sequelae of the transference topic in the article before, Kemper basically tells the patient that he's homosexual only if the analyst says he is.

A new journal can renew psychoanalysis in Germany only by foregrounding work undertaken and composed by supporters of Freud's science during the Third Reich. In his introduction to the first issue of *Zeitschrift für Psychoanalyse* Müller-Braunschweig furthermore suggests that it was for political reasons that the articles had to wait until 1949 to appear. But the centerpiece in the foreground that's deemed essential to the new journal's mission, "Beginn einer Analyse" (The Beginning of an Analysis), was originally Werner Kemper's 1938 presentation before a gathering of adherents of the separate but to-be-coordinated psychodynamic approaches. When was it written up as an article? Kemper's current address on the page is Rio de Janeiro.

Müller-Braunschweig explains in his editorial note that Kemper was trying to initiate a mutual understanding among the different schools via his practical account of the start of treatment. Kemper's own "introduction" (not published in the journal but from which Müller-Braunschweig cites) addressed the lexical impasse that results when pseudo-differences and pseudo-similarities arise around the same terms. That's why his presentation is focused on observation. The only theoretical term Kemper uses and situates is transference.

The transference topic gets introduced via the iconic couch, which gives a sense of the setting of his presentation. He introduces the couch through his own innovation in the setting of "classical" analysis.[4] He prefers to sit to the side of the couch (and not behind it) so the patient can see him when he wishes to but otherwise sees no one when looking straight ahead and into the middle distance. Kemper's own flexibility is his license to observe that sitting across from one another interpersonally eye to eye is an obstacle to the transference, which is intrapsychic. The basic facet of the transference is that the patient brings it to session, reanimating and recycling pathogenic experiential material, which led to the development of the neurosis in the first place (8). That's why it's closely linked to resistance: you can't treat with it, and you can't treat without it. The patient projects onto the analyst all the early imagines of parents, siblings, the housekeeper, and – Kemper adds before the etc. – teachers, who are already party to the majority fare of transference relations. The intrapsychic past swabs over onto the setting of the session.

When Kemper asks that he begin by reporting what's crossing his mind, the patient responds hesitantly that the white doorframe like in a hospital makes an uncanny impression. Kemper is quick to point out that he went to great lengths to make sure his office decor was homey and not clinical. But then the patient recalls the earlier situation: in his boyhood he suffered from a lung ailment, convalescing at home and in a sort of sanitarium. It turned out not to be anything serious. He suffered mainly under his mother's exaggerated care. This is the first loose thread that gives Kemper something to tug at.

Not until you are reading the article does anyone know or want to know that the presenting problem at the start of this analysis is homosexuality. Kemper however lists it in third place: "Furthermore he senses on occasion a very disturbing homosexual impulse in the form of fantasies of an imperative nature" (7). A patient who presents the problem of his homosexuality even though he's not says more about the German culture of psychoanalysis that continued through the Third Reich than it does about what afflicts him.

Admittedly the declared homosexuality of Kemper's patient is more dread desire than practice, but the patient feels his marriage is in jeopardy. After one and a half years, four sessions per week, the treatment succeeds in good measure because Kemper does not tackle the problem directly. Indeed, he ignores the patient's wish to stick to the presenting problem and its cure, which he sees as the obstacle during treatment. Instead, Kemper identifies in the masque of his patient's cultured disposition denial of conflict with his father. Kemper guides the patient to drop his mask of submissiveness, which his mother imposed, and restore the phallic interest he showed in childhood, which his mother couldn't abide. The lung ailment that even kept him out of military service during World War One had been the mother's opportunity to render her son harmless.

Kemper observes that when the patient says "mother" he is non-verbally ill at ease, like he's trying to rebutton his jacket and isn't sure whether he skipped a row. Kemper asks him what was going on in his mind during the pantomime. Instead of answering, he tries to continue, but when "mother" comes up again, he must go on with the show. The third time it happens Kemper interprets. Oh, he's buttoned up alright: up tight. The patient responds with more backstory.

Before the season of maternal care, he had been a wild child, even throwing an open pocketknife at his brother, "etc." "But none of that is important, why am I talking about it, I'm here because of the homosexuality" (9). You can tell that Kemper is acquiescing but unimpressed when, reluctantly, he gives the floor to the patient who lists the ingredients of his homosexual makeup. The patient had a schoolboy crush on his cousin, and they exchanged kisses. Not so long ago when he was a student, he had a thing for a former Guard Cuirassier, and it came to genital contact ("genitale Berührungen"). Since then, he has been "damned to homosexuality." When he sees cute boys ("schmucke Jungen"), he cannot calm himself (9).

Next session the patient bursts in with his worries that Kemper was put off last time. He could tell by the analyst's hesitant handshake at the end of the session, not firm like at the start. Kemper says he wasn't aware of a change and suggests they see what turns up, whether his impression might have been a projection (9–10). Kemper is the one, the only one who can give him a hand with his problem (10). Silence.

Last night the patient had an odd dream illuminating two settings in one, his single bona fide homosexual experience as well as his analysis. Together with fellow Cuirassiers he is captured by a revolutionary horde. The leader of the mob, who has a moustache and is uncanny like a Dostoevsky figure, wants to force the patient to swear allegiance to the republican constitution. But he has already sworn fealty to his king (10). During association with elements of the dream, he remembers that although he didn't serve in the war owing to his alleged lung ailment, he was enlisted in 1918 to work in the *Ordnungsdienst*, the organization maintaining public order. He was stationed in Berlin and at the outbreak of the revolution a mob did enter the barracks to celebrate and fraternize with them. The intruders brought along their women. It was a gruesomely uninhibited horde, drinking, shouting, whoring. There were Cuirassiers in his corps, including the one with whom he was once intimate (10).

The dream scene is by 1938 a Nazi propaganda motif. Leftist heteros vulgarize the ideals of fraternity. The homosocial withdrawal of the pure in heart counts as a positive attribute, even if it does border on the taboo of homosexuality. Overcoming the circle jerk phase in candidates immune to left-leaning sexual freedom is what makes the treatment of homosexuality eminently believable and desirable. Explicitly supported, even ordered by the authorities, it is one of the three foci at the institute for the coordination of the working groups.[5] The other two are improving efficiency in the workplace and the treatment of war neurosis. Kemper's case in fact double dips, since the alleged lung ailment that converted the wild child to his homosocial adaptation kept him out of the war like another shell shock victim or malingerer. The mother's influence isn't all wrong since it did keep her boy from joining the leftist gangbangers. Kemper succeeds in recalibrating the good citizen in his patient, making room for enough phallic wildness to penetrate reproduction. At the conclusion Kemper extols the patient's improvement in his work, too. A triple dip success story.

Kemper asks about the Dostoevsky reference in the dream. The interrogation scene in *Crime and Punishment* is, for the patient, about the criminal not knowing whether the prosecutor is asking his questions with any foreknowledge. "This dialogue diabolically balances upon the blade of the knife, *that* is what is so uncanny" (10). In other words, Kemper says, someone with a bad conscience fears that in conversation he can be seen through. Even when the patient admits that the moustache is like Kemper's, he still doesn't know what the analyst wants to make of the dream; it all makes sense, but he just doesn't feel it (11). What was hot was that the man with the moustache wanted to force the patient to exchange vows with vulgar heterosexuality. The missing piece that Kemper is after is that the patient is only pretending to be emo homosexual.

Are you my prisoner? Kemper asks (11). The patient does the pantomime number that "mother" otherwise triggers. By now the word doesn't have to be uttered to produce the effect. He surrenders information he withheld during all those sessions of interrogation and torture. When Kemper's housekeeper opened the door, the patient was reminded of his mother. Her apron's shoulder strap had slipped down, and he flashed on his topless mother, espied when at age four or five he entered the master bedroom unannounced. Every homosexual was a vulgar heterosexual in childhood.

His mother saw no problem, but he was thoroughly shocked and ran away. To this day he can't kiss his mother and when he visits home and spends the night, he must be sure that there is one empty room between their bedrooms. The wife is that empty bedroom. So, it was the patient who felt guilty about his buttoned lips, which he projected as Kemper handing him a limp rag, the charge left dangling since he threw down the gauntlet: homosexuality or no father, I mean farther.

His patient's view of the world is painted in soft pastels; there are no distinct black-and-white divides, but only soft gray; there are no dissonances, no profanity (13). His voice is carefully modulated, pleasingly fluent. His affect is dialed down, evened out. Like his language, like his attire, like his character – so is his sexuality. He's mild-mannered with his wife, always looking after her wishes, never making demands in a masculine manner, seeing her not as a woman (not even as a whore) but as the holy mother.

Next session he wants to know how Kemper profiling him as soft and submissive contributes anything at all to understanding the problem at hand, the problem of homosexuality (13). Last night he had a homosexual dream (14). He's standing in front of the theater with his cousin, his crush from early adolescence. A policeman is even there, but they don't care. Their intimacies culminate in mutual masturbation. Then they go their separate ways while grinning cynically at the cop. The patient can go no further via association whether with the dream as a whole or in any of its parts. Kemper can't do anything with it: the defiant gesture, he says, is not convincing. Yes, there is something missing, the other dream from last night. In that dream he was supposed to give an entertaining and amusing talk. Suddenly he has the idea to act as though the microphone weren't on yet, and converse in a casual and relaxed way with the colleague standing next to him. The audience falls for it, finding it a riot to be involuntary witness to a private exchange. That's the patient all right, pretending to be casual, aiming only for the effect on his audience. Yes, a man seated in the front row looked like Kemper. "He grasps and formulates it himself. The mask is the mainstay of his character" (14). This is the breakthrough toward which Kemper was guiding his patient.

His mother imposed the mask, religiously installing in her son identification with Christ, which he carries forward as the masque of softness and submissiveness. At the time of its introduction, however, the growing identification was attended by fantasies of being tormented by his father (15). The conflict with the father returns in the transference.

The patient brings to session a dream in which he visits a vulgarly appointed abode that's clearly a caricature of Kemper's apartment and office (14). The staff is boorish and loose. A kitschy painting that hangs over the office desk, however, doesn't correspond to anything in Kemper's place. But the patient proudly identifies it. It's a landscape his father painted (15). At this very moment in the session, he suddenly realizes that the painting is dismal, which in German can be conveyed by what the patient cries out, calling it a "ham" (*Schinken*). The idealization of his father as an admirable, morally upright, spiritually elevated person of culture was one big ham job. This change in the patient's understanding of his father, of the paternal relation, leads directly to the dissolution of the "homosexuality" Kemper now floats in quotes.

Notes

1 Käthe Dräger, "Bemerkungen zu den Zeitumständen und zum Schicksal der Psychoanalyse und der Psychotherapie in Deutschand zwischen 1933 und 1949," *PSYCHE*, 4, 25 (April 1971), 255–268.

2 Werner Kemper, "Die Übertragung. Ihre diagnostischen und therapeutischen Möglichkeiten," *Zeitschrift für Psychoanalyse. Unter Mitwirkung von Psychoanalytikern des In- und Auslands*, ed. Carl Müller-Braunschweig, vol. 1, no. 2 (1949/1950), 99–121.

The information on the article's original status as a report in Nazi Berlin is given in the note on p. 99. Page references are given in the text.

3 A few months later, on a lecture tour through the United States, Künkel decided at the outbreak of the war to stay in Los Angeles where he soon had his own institute. But his second wife and colleague, still in Berlin, took care not to give a political spin to his separation from Germany throughout the war.

4 Werner Kemper, "Beginn einer Analyse," *Zeitschrift für Psychoanalyse*, 1, 1 (1949), 7–16; here: 8. The subsequent page references are given in the text.

5 Hans-Martin Lohmann and Lutz Rosenkötter, "Psychoanalyse in Hitlerdeutschland. Wie war es wirklich?" in *Psychoanalyse und Nationalsozialismus. Beträge zur Bearbeitung eines unbewältigten Traumas*, ed. Hans-Martin Lohmann (Frankfurt a/M: Fischer Taschenbuch Verlag, 1984), 54–77. The research foci at the institute are succinctly presented in section VI.

Chapter 11

Lady MacKemper

I postponed looking at an earlier case example Kemper provided in his presentation on the transference, reserving it to forge a segue to the setting of the secret, not the secret of his betrayal of Rittmeister, but the secret of his outlandish machinations on behalf of his wife's wish to be a didactic psychoanalyst. The article on the transference, published a decade after it was presented, already gives Kemper's address: Rio de Janeiro. It's the case example of an OCD patient who three weeks into treatment is revealed in session to be oppressed, uncomfortable, almost guilty. Neither Kemper nor his patient can comprehend this shift in mood within the total situation (104).

> That evening my wife mentions in passing that she met the new patient for the first time on his way to my office. Since I know by the patient's description that the one woman who played a role in his life must resemble my wife, I bring it up to the patient in the next session, in which his mood is still oppressed, asking why he didn't mention encountering my wife. (104)

What does that have to do with his illness and treatment?! Then after a long silence he opens a chapter of the history he had omitted. When he saw Kemper's wife he flashed on a fantasy of sexual violence, which tortured him, but which he immediately forgot. Now that the fantasy is back, however, it begins to bring back early childhood memories of his slightly older sister. He stops short and bursts out: now I remember everything! He was in treatment with one of Kemper's colleagues for over two years but then had to stop because that man too had a wife who triggered the dread fantasies. At the same time, he broke off relations with the woman he was seeing, the one and only in his life.

> If I hadn't been so rigorous in finding out about his encounter with my wife, the patient would probably have run away tortured by his overwhelming fantasies. At the very least I would have lost a very important and for the patient an extremely impressive point of access to a key position of his neurosis – much to the patient's detriment. (105)

DOI: 10.4324/9781003797708-14

I agree with Hans Füchner that Kemper's 1964 article, "Die Doppelgesichtigkeit von Tatbeständen" (The Two Faces of Facts),[1] evinces an analytic-empathic understanding of the psychic injury that leads a victim of the Third Reich to apply for compensation, a claim Kemper had been called in to assess or rather reassess. In the third sentence summarizing the inevitable misunderstanding between a petitioner seeking compensation and the appraiser, Kemper refers to an unconscious or undeclared expectation of "a type of *Wiedergutmachung* (reparation)" (546).[2] In the opening reflections on the situation of evaluating applicants for restitution, in which Kemper marks the actual demand for *Wiedergutmachung* as impossible and unconscious, he allows that he can go no further here with this problem because the topic of his article is instead the "double-facedness" of the facts (548). Kemper is hopeful that psychosomatic medicine, which is now making inroads in Central Europe, can help in understanding the entirety of what really happened to the patient applying for compensation.

After Frau N. was turned down in 1957, the United Restitution Organization of Rio de Janeiro referred her case to Kemper. A first reading of her file convinces Kemper that the judgments of his two predecessors make sense in the setting of worker's compensation. But in the sessions with Frau N., particularly the third one, he understands what the injury in fact is and that it qualifies. Up to this turning point, the case looked like thousands of pension applications following work-related accidents and their evaluation in terms of consequent reduction of the capacity for work. Frau N. based her claim on the interrelation between her physical injuries, one occurring at the forced labor camp, the other while exiting the tram shortly after liberation. However, no causal connection could be seen to obtain nor was her ability to work more than minimally reduced in the course of both accidents and the physical injuries. That was the judgment of the first two evaluators.

The first injury happened toward the end of 1943, "a time when the war had already entered its catastrophic final phase."

> The "total solution" of the Jewish problem (*Judenproblem*), in other words, the systematic mass annihilation, had been decided and the corresponding executions were already being carried out in a major way. Against this world-historical background accidents befalling a Jewish inmate of a forced labor camp… meant, even when the injury was minor, certain extinction if the ability to work was at all compromised. (553)

This is pronounced in plain text with an equanimity that is to Kemper's credit.

She was able to hide the first injury with the help of her brother, who treated her wounds so no cause for diminishment of her capacity for work would show. Later, when she was transferred to Auschwitz and then to Bergen-Belsen, she had to pass the opening inspection that separated those who were still able to work from the majority sent to the gas chamber. The patient had already lost her mother in this selection setting. Kemper spells it out: the medically justified determination that her physical wound was minor misses the context completely.

The second injury that happened when she fell getting off the tram in 1945 was rejected outright by the earlier evaluators for being the fault alone of her own carelessness. But the backstory to this second accident packs the bigger wallop, as Kemper discovers. A few days before the French liberated the camp, Frau N. learned from newly arrived Jewish workers the location of the facility where her brother was "employed." Because of her weakened condition she waited two weeks to recover her basic strength before heading out to reunite with him. On her way at last she heard that just prior to the arrival of the Allied forces mass executions of forced laborers had taken place. And just before she arrives the news reaches her that the workers at her brother's address were machine-gunned down. Feeling faint, she falls while exiting the tram.

There's a "continuity error" here because the news that makes her fall had stated that there was an exception. One laborer survived by playing dead. How come everyone (not only Frau N. but also Kemper) assumes that the survivor couldn't be her brother? Why is the exception on record and yet ignored? Frau N. immediately occupies the state of exception, partakes of the metabolic low point of playing dead and takes the fall for her own sole survival. The continuity error lodged in Kemper's study represents, as always, unacknowledged and unmournable loss. The patient's fall (*Sturz*) in 1945 is redoubled by Kemper's own misprision – his obedient, dutiful, cursory reading of Frau N.'s file. "In reading the earlier statements I pounced on… the facts (*stürzte ich mich auf die... Tatbestände*)." The doubling of Frau N.'s fall (*Sturz*) in 1945 confirms Kemper's recognition that he had gone about it all wrong, reading at first only one of the faces of the facts. He had been in cahoots with the way the patient's declarations in session were dictated by her preference for physical factors. That's why Kemper believes her: she doesn't know the true value of her statements in their third session.

Heretofore she clearly felt diverted from her purpose whenever Kemper questioned her on, to her mind, unrelated matters. She responded curtly and reluctantly. The more fluent exchanges during the earlier evaluation were only possible because they talked past one another. Kemper sees the patient holding onto the leg injuries as the visible graspable symbol of all that she and her loved ones had suffered. I would specify that it's her brother somewhere between dead and playing dead who's still caring for her wounds in secret.

Around the double *Sturz* we learn that the patient has all along been complicit with the cursory view of her physical complaint and its physical causation. Why, now that he sees what she doesn't see, does it cross his mind – even though he quickly dismisses the thought – that she's exaggerating? Kemper updates the concept of neurosis current in the earlier evaluations, which he identifies as vintage 1926 and in which constitutional factors were emphasized (557). Adherence to this old view leaves out the changes that psychosomatic medicine has brought about in the meantime in the understanding of neurosis. Any latency notwithstanding, what's decisive are the environmental factors that are traumatic enough to cause neurosis. The distinction between disposition and environment no longer holds.

That psychic injury can yield physical symptoms is as old as hysteria and is the background for the analytic understanding of shell shock or war neurosis that led ultimately to the continued centrality of Freud's science amidst the psychotherapies even at the Nazi Berlin Institute. Kemper pounces upon strands of "new" research in order to network for his return to Germany, which he was already planning.[3] By the end of the article, which opened with the view that medical progress in Central Europe was behind international advances in psychosomatic medicine, he sets himself up by listing and annotating German practitioners who were equally allied with the new import of psychosomatic symptomatology, particularly in the evaluations of PTSD victims of the Nazi era. None of the names belong to the institute where Kemper once worked except J.H. Schultz, whose autogenic training was by then the main export of postwar German psychotherapy. Kemper's gesture also participates in hiding the back story of the star of West German psychoanalysis, Alexander Mitscherlich. Coming out of psychosomatic medicine, which was in fact first introduced in Germany, Mitscherlich professed to be coming out of the return of psychoanalysis. At the forefront of this return Kemper joined Mitscherlich in facing a hidden past as the future of a new analytic interface for identifying the psychic reality in the zomboid ailments of the survivors of the death camps.

Kemper could escape his wife's ongoing imposture in Brazil only by returning to Germany. What had been going on for years was beginning to undermine him: he had dutifully and unprofessionally supported her every claim to be a licensed German analyst, even training analyst.[4] It was clear that she needed a stage other than his institute but at the same time she stalwartly insisted on remaining a member in good standing. A crisis point in the conflict between her demands and the opposition of Kemper's colleagues was reached around the time he was the third evaluator assessing Frau N.'s compensation claim. It was at this time that members of the psychoanalytic institute that Kemper had founded and was still directing pressed against Anna Kattrin Kemper the charge of falsifying her credentials. She first joined the society as a licensed graphologist (which she was) and then upgraded to analyst, indeed training analyst (which was invention). As we saw, Besserman Vianna is stuck on Cabernite's recourse to graphology as though it were the biggest clue in tracking the Nazi transmission. The secret that no one must tell touches on the CV of A.K. Kemper, one that her husband's former Berlin colleagues, who knew her socially as W. Kemper's wife, conspired to invent and corroborate.

The complaints lodged against the director's wife did occasion a 1962 site visit organized by the International Society. The illustrious committee (Robert D. Knight, Leon Grinberg, and Bertram D. Lewin) that flew down to Rio was charged with investigating the allegations or, more likely, with assuaging the strife that was bad publicity for the fledgling tributary of psychoanalysis in Brazil. Although it was recommended that Frau Kemper take refresher tutorials with Marie Langer, the committee basically accepted all her forged documents as being in order.

While pursuing graphology as the leading signifier of the encrypted Kemper secret,[5] Besserman Vianna works through the thicket of the influence of Lady MacKemper, whose life in Besserman Vianna's book is cut short seven years earlier than her actual death date (201). In making recourse to a graphologist to identify her handwriting in the note to Langer, Besserman Vianna sees Cabernite occupying the position of his analytic father's wife (204). If Rittmeister was still Kemper's didactic analysand at the time of his arrest, then the training analysis had been going on for five years, which Besserman Vianna underscores was a mysteriously long relationship especially for those times (190). But only by agreeing with Cocks that Erna Göring must have told Kemper about the investigation of Rittmeister can she breach the graphology impasse and address the first generation of the secret (191). There is no corroboration whatsoever, cryptonymically or criminologically, that Kemper was privy to any information that made him complicit in Rittmeister's downfall.

Around the kernel of her graphology license, A.K. Kemper could have spun the profile of an analytic or psychodynamic therapist, but that wasn't good enough for her. She wanted to be a psychoanalyst recognized by the International Society. That's why after she was able with the help of her husband to wring letters out of Felix Boehm substantiating her alleged activities as analytic candidate prior to the move to Brazil, she dropped his support once Müller Braunschweig's new organization, the DPV, had been certified by the International Association.

In 1951 she applied for membership as analyst in the DPV based on the documentation she had extracted from Boehm and the evaluations that Schultz-Hencke and J.H. Schultz supplied quite willingly. She traveled to Berlin to deliver the lecture and pass the inspection for membership. The lecture was found acceptable but not the discussion that ensued, which she flunked. Müller Braunschweig had to disappoint her husband, explaining in a letter just how deplorably unprepared she had been.

Why didn't A.K. Kemper go all out and claim a start as analytic candidate before 1933? Because many members of the Jewish majority at the Institute back then were available in the postwar world as witnesses to her false testimony? Apparently, that's what the ambiguous continued existence of analysis in Nazi Berlin was good for – as a quarry for piecing together false credentials. In 1933 she started out as Kemper's secretary working on her M.R.S.[6] Rittmeister in his prison diaries mentions that he should have secured his marriage with children the way Kemper had done. She bore him three sons in swift succession but already in 1936 found time to train as a graphologist. Like going to art school, studying graphology in Nazi Germany did not require a successfully concluded secondary school education.

When her husband returned to West Germany, the society got rid of her or, rather, she left before she could be thrown out. She established with her coterie of supporters several psychoanalytic associations, including a clinic, and became Kattrin the Great for her followers. When she conducted Couples Therapy in groups there were over one hundred participants. But Kattrin wasn't even her given name, which is why its exact spelling – by others, her husband or even by her – fluctuated to such a degree. Her story qualifies as another "Tale of Misogyny" by Patricia Highsmith not by dint of her being so driven and destructive but because the men back in Germany all so readily conspired to corroborate her hysterical claim that she had been a successful analytic candidate in Nazi Berlin, something they would never have done for a man. If this could be restaged as an allegorical pageant, A.K. Kemper, aka Kattrin the Great, would be the figurehead captioning for all to see and read imposture as the inheritance of Nazi psychoanalysis.

Although a psychoanalyst hearing her claim to be a born analyst might identify a narcissistic disorder, there were many who felt she was right to think of herself a natural talent in psychotherapy. The corroborating anecdote she liked to tell in support of this predisposition concerned her little untreatable patient, Maria. After their session the child was being bullied by another patient. When Frau Kemper saw that Maria was on the floor crying, she rushed over, clasped her to her bosom and comforted her. A connection was made at this turning point that Frau Kemper was able to see through to Maria's cure.

W. Kemper finally didn't want to go down for, with or through Lady MacKemper, who kept urging him to more and more outrageous falsifications on behalf of her talent-driven career, and so, within three years of the article about the double *Sturz* (I hear an echo of the tall tale of Maria) he closed his twenty-year Rio de Janeiro chapter, divorced her, and departed. He died two years after Marie Langer made the Lobo-Cabernite Affair a public scandal. But for Kemper the scandal he left behind was A.K. Kemper's pop analytic career in the place where he was forgotten, but where many would come to remember him as the Nazi.

One of his early didactic analysands, Galina Schneider, argued that there were two crises that compromised Kemper's Brazilian career. The first was his controversial appointment of A.K. Kemper as training analyst at his institute, the second, which the first crisis introduced and prepared for, was the Lobo-Cabernite scandal.[7] Schneider characterizes Kemper's administrative style as firm but not authoritarian. However, that changed when he imposed his wife on bona fide analysts as their colleague. Besserman Vianna writes that when Werner Kemper was criticized in 1951 for enthroning his wife, he struck out against Burke, calling him insane (198). That would put the blame for the rift that led to the doubling of the analytic institute in Rio and came so tendentiously close to a World War Two profile of the contestants as perpetrator and victim, on Kemper's because-I-say-so insistence that his wife's wish for membership in the institute be fulfilled. Besserman-Vianna sees A.K. Kemper as the bum steer. But the graphology that she does attend to in her reading just isn't the thread leading through the labyrinthine condition of the husband's encryptment of his Nazi past or his past in Nazi Berlin.

To be sure, a certain resoluteness, even ruthlessness in decision making was carried over into Cabernite's handling of the second crisis. In Kemper's defense Schneider underscores that he was forced to multitask roles that are rarely combined all in one person. Her account brought one of the Kemper sons, Jochen, to the fore of commentary. He dismisses her tendentious characterization of his mother as well as her allusion to marital conflict leading to his father returning to Berlin. But by adding another crisis he underscores Schneider's point about his father occupying too many positions of respect. He was at once didactic analyst, supervisor, instructor and director as well as founder of international psychoanalysis in Rio de Janeiro. In 1953 Kemper was arrested on charges submitted by mental health professionals outside the institute that he was engaged in illegal activities as a medical doctor. As the multi-occupied and cathected founding father Kemper attracted, and his son Jochen knows enough to supply the litany, transference conflicts, Oedipal and sibling rivalries, neurotic repetition compulsions and other unconscious mechanisms.[8]

Kemper's secret was that he exploited the imposture of a saved German psychoanalysis on his better half's behalf and ruthlessly imposed a counterfeit analyst on his duly certified colleagues.

Everything we unpacked around the false lead of graphology, including the outrageous career moves of Katrin Kemper, is set up as well in Besserman Vianna's book. But the authoritarian manner Kemper flexed on his wife's behalf is a cultural difference and a dead stop, I submit, in the alleged itinerary of the crypt.

In *The Cabinet of Doctor Caligari*, the first crime on the range of the occult belongs to the German psychopathology of everyday life. The bureaucrat who denies the doctor a permit does so with a rudeness that the German law protective of its bureaucracy (punishing any client who insults a state employee) catches on the rebound. At the start of my stay in Germany, I published readings in *Germany: A Science Fiction* weighing the integration of the World War Two foe against the continued bias among the former Allies against all things German. At the end of my time in Germany, I can offer an anecdotal character psychology of the Germans illuminated by their relationship to the offices and authorities of state management. Like Highsmith in France, in Berlin I came to know my share of difficulties with the tax authorities. It's not so much that the authorities were in the wrong, but the overriding power structure hypnotizes the competence of the German tax advisers whose often clueless efforts on your behalf invite the audit that's waiting to happen. Like a sorry version of *The Castle*, the authoritarian actionism of Hegel's universal class infantilizes the whole slew of intermediaries and assistants until their mediating realm of representation becomes as essential as it is worthless.

When I told a thoroughly pleasant and civilized Berlin merchant about my difficulties, which was why there was a delay in paying him, he responded charmingly that the German civil service was a cosmos of its own. Another empathic German friend offered comfort in the form of an analogy. The unpleasantness of dealing with a German state agency was like putting up with the rash in your face, which is bound to go away once the causative agent is again remote. When it was in your face you just had to get through it. Why should anyone whose relationship to the German bureaucracy isn't a birthright hang around for more of the same? I came to understand the remark that I at first only found insulting, namely that no foreigner voluntarily resides in Germany who isn't of German descent.

That the German people were under the threat of Nazi standards is the maverick insight of Andreas Peglau in his study of Wilhelm Reich's banishment in the setting of adjusting psychoanalysis to survive in the Third Reich. I add to it that the native condition of getting through the business with bureaucracy is the rehearsal for and repetition of this torture. National Socialism raised the bar on adjusting to the administered state by treating the Germans, on average, as the allergens. The Nazi attack on European Jewry was leveled in the first place against Jews who were Germans. The Nazis wanted to protect and project more than just being Aryan. Next in store for shoring up the psychic status quo was sorting out figures of protracted care without a cure in sight.

Willingness to view any contradiction as neurotic, the bedrock of the Göring Institute's success story, valorizes psychotherapy as the guarantor of life-changing, life-saving cures. The pure cure guides the all-out effort to secure it in advance of neurotic mediation by determining the choice of partners in marriage and reproduction. Increasingly, a norm beyond the ken of therapy was being installed, one that called many Germans into question – for being odd, eccentric, shy and bashful, too intellectual, the loner type, and so on. While in the military setting oddballs were therapeutically integrated for the exercise in finitude, on the home front an inscrutable norm was pronouncing a curse upon German existence.

We can say that eugenics was upheld by National Socialism as its psy-fi reality test. That sacrifices had to be made to guarantee the viability of purity was not restricted to the sessions of therapists and patients. It was no secret that the geographical and historical situation of Germany (the Thirty Years' War!) had mixed a certain measure of foreignness into the bloodlines, which meant that, by and large, only good enough Aryans were available. Your average German therefore passed as Aryan through constant trials of reevaluation that were hell bent on identifying untreatable character defects.

In "Some Psychodynamic Factors Behind Tensions That Cause Wars," John Rickman, the UK analyst whose 1946 site visit to Berlin helps organize our visit with the psychoanalysts who remained in Germany after 1933, gives a World-War-Two example of projection.

> Hitler and those who accepted his ideas projected their hate beyond the frontier and imagined that Germany was beset with enemies, even at a time when in fact her neighbours were friendly. Once the projection process is underway a vicious circle is established. Now what was originally hated? It was Germany itself, but there were also feelings of good regard for the motherland. As the conflict was intolerable, a solution was reached by turning the hate outwards.[9]

The same holds true for the mother tongue in the Third Reich. Honoring and elevating the language, lifting and separating it from all the collateral evidence of High German's indebtedness to translation, the Nazis loved German to death.

Peglau and Rickman are justified in their view, paradoxically perhaps, by a counter strain in German national character psychology. In this study, I am reclaiming, carefully I hope, what's usually written off as a dangerous ideology of phrases. German culture spawned this genre of psychological understanding as though it were its own owner's manual. I aim this canon in the direction of allegory and keep turning it around throughout the study not as proof but like a prop in the pageant of self-understanding (or rationalization) that underlies the overall opportunism and imposture of the German analysts. In addition, then, to the ability to get through the controlling interest the bureaucracy takes in you and your goods, which exemplifies the German availability for finding one's way around a bad situation, we can add that there is a preoccupation with protecting the soul strains of the Germans, for which those in the outside world don't have, as we say in Berlin, an organ. There is also this inner trajectory to the German National Character's quarrel with the world.

There is honesty in dog stories. Those in charge of establishing the Weimaraner breed in the late nineteenth century formed an exclusive club for maintaining the stock and ensuring that responsible owners would oversee its development. Only club members were entitled to adopt Weimaraner. In 1929, Howard Knight, an American sportsman, was the first outsider allowed to join the German club and take two dogs to his foreign land. The German club members were so protective of their sensitive Weimaraner that they first sent Knight two desexed dogs. Knight was not deterred and kept right on applying to receive foundation dogs for breeding in the US. In 1938, he finally acquired three females and a male puppy. In 1942 there was an American Weimaraner club. Born in 1943, German American photographer William Wegman provided the happy ending to this story in the series of portraits of Weimaraner role playing human subjects.

The international dog training language may still be German, but the history of the Weimaraner breed doesn't transmit a continuity from Germany to the US. While in the US a one-big-happy-family model pertains in parks where humans of all ages and their dogs comingle, in Germany dogs cannot be brought to a children's playground and children are disallowed at dog parks. The German segregation is a wise precaution that sides with the sensitivity of the animal. My dog Elli was terrified of children and barked at all of them, a big problem in the US. On a street in Berlin when we had to get past a little girl walking with her father and Elli started barking up a storm it was the father who scolded his daughter for carelessly provoking a reaction that was understandable. There was a place for us that didn't endanger canine odd balls.

The profiled eccentrics in line for Nazi bullying were recognizable through a certain German tolerance for emo-adolescent variations on the schizoid's outsider status. German literature lets loners be without punishment or redemption. What is more important than the dictates of any norm in the psychological sense is the requirement of being registered, identified and ultimately protected. This is where the two strains of German national character psychology meet, giving the bureaucracy a measure of control over the benign strain of a German knack for eccentricity.

Something so obvious that it cannot be readily comprehended is that no other culture in which I have spent quality time has shown a happier ambivalence toward homosexuality. After an extended stay in West Berlin in the 1980s I was making my departure from the building in which I had resided for the duration when I for the first time recognized that the woman once again mopping the floor at the foot of the stairwell was the trans wife of the concierge. You would think that the POV of neighbors marking or overlooking an oddity would have guided my recognition months earlier, but there was no perspective of intolerance brought to bear. My parting shot of recognition was the first time I saw her up close, right in front of me. Was I the first one to disturb the idyll with a double take? Should I not be allowed to adopt a Weimaraner?

Notes

1 Werner Kemper, "*Die Doppelgesichtigkeit von Tatbeständen. Zur Begutachtung von Entschädigungsansprüchen wegen nationalsozialisticher Verfolgung,*" *PSYCHE*, 9 (1964), 546–560. Page references are given in the text.
2 Since the early years of Konrad Adenauer's chancellorship, the key term in the lingua franca of the postwar West German business of making reparation for the crimes of the Third Reich was *Wiedergutmachung*. The way the policy was set up, any damage done by the Nazi persecution to the ability to work and carry out a life's plan and intended job description qualifies for restitution or compensation. I argued in *Germany: A Science Fiction* that this formulation of a wider ranging comprehension of the damage done in terms of the right to work was dictated by the limited ability to identify empathically during the first phase of recovery from a psychopathic state. But importantly it represents for this population healing from violence, including their own, a step toward repair, which moves closer to the onset of the ability to mourn.
3 Just the same it is an ambivalent adjustment since what awaited him in West Germany was the ruling influence of Alexander Mitscherlich, who came out of psychosomatic medicine before he caught up with his reputation and became a psychoanalyst. Kemper doubly ignores Mitscherlich by forgetting his mentor Viktor von Weizsäcker, whose psychosomatic research was already in place in the Third Reich. Central Europe didn't have to wait for this research to arrive from abroad.
4 My knowledge of the case of Anna Kattrin Kemper comes from Hans Füchner's thoroughgoing documentation of it: "'Fremdartiger bunter Vogel' oder 'Große Dame der Psychoanalyse'? Zur atypischen Berufsbiographie von Anna Kattrin Kemper" ("Strange colorful bird" or "Grande Dame of Psychoanalysis"? On the Atypical Career Biography of Anna Kattrin Kemper), *Psychoanalyse.lu* (October 2011), 1–31. This is an online version of its publication in *Luzifer-Amor*, 39, 20 (2007), 80–118.
5 As late as her Estates General lecture in 2000 Besserman Vianna refers to the graphologist Cabernite asked to perform the handwriting test as "a technician employed by an agency of the military government" (p. 5 of the online document). That Harald Schultz-Hencke's mother was the first woman to command and practice graphology in Berlin either rings true in the corner with Kemper's secret or brings down Besserman Vianna's construction of Kemper's guilt. Graphology isn't restricted to crime investigation, which is how Cabernite used it. Ludwig Klages reinforced handwriting analysis as a serious facet of eclectic psychotherapy. Another member of the Stefan George circle, Klages was part of the linguistic change that came over academic discourse. In promoting expression, Klage's poetic prose with its vocabulary of synonyms competed with the acronymic secret handshake of jargon, bringing to a head the rejection of jargon and idiom on behalf of something more complete, more like a language. He however kept his distance from the Nazis.
6 Wolfgang Bock is alone in referring to Kattrin Kemper as Werner Kemper's former patient.
7 Galina Schneider, "Stellungnahme zu 'Traurige Psychotropen' von Hans Füchner," *PSYCHE*, 39 (July 1985), 1133–1149.
8 "Brief von Jochen Kemper an die Psychoanalytische Gesellschaft von Rio de Janeiro (SPRJ)," *PSYCHE*, 42 (July 1988), 1016–1020; here: 1019.
9 *No Ordinary Psychoanalyst: The Exceptional Contributions of John Rickman*, ed. Pearl King (London and New York: Karnak Books, 2003), 246–247.

Part Three

The Colleagues at the Göring Institute

Chapter 12

B&B

Felix Boehm and Carl Müller Braunschweig inherited by hook and by crook the psychoanalytic institute in Berlin from Jewish colleagues who might have been the better choice for its administration. But the Jewish members had to go and had to go willingly. Following that sorry negotiation for the acquiescence of their former confederates in their own exclusion, the duo participated in the opening series of the transmogrification of the psychoanalytic institute and the German psychoanalytic society allegedly to save Freud's science. Werner Kemper's career escalated in the vacuum, but he was still a generation or so younger than those two and had to wait his turn. To situate and introduce John Rittmeister we already indicated that Boehm and Müller-Braunschweig were necessarily to some degree double agents since – and this can't be emphasized enough – Freud was still alive, and they owed fealty to him.

No one up or down the ranks of international analysis seemed to care much for Boehm, but he was a local celeb by dint of the notoriety he cultivated.[1] A Baltic German like Alfred Rosenberg, he had a combative nature, which he styled with flippant and outrageous remarks. Studying Ian Fleming's style of thought comprising the world of James Bond, I could observe how even slight knowledge of psychoanalysis suffices to present racist and sexist opinion as dialectically bound to or by the unconscious – en route, in other words, to real insight. While still a Freudian, Jung excelled at apodictic reversals of opposition of race or gender in interviews he gave during his US tours. We can imagine Boehm, who liked to boast that the legs of his female patients were improving under analysis,[2] in the role of a Bond antagonist (or distorted double). When John Rickman was sent to Berlin to assess the five analysts who stuck it out at the Göring Institute his documentation of the meeting with Boehm shows that he was immune to the Blofeld style of diversion (perhaps because he was a Quaker):

> He praised the Americans, denounced the Russians, and showed his lack of tact and underlying hostility by asking me if I, as an Englishman, could explain why it was the German women despised the British troops. They were cold and frigid sexually and hadn't the spunk of the Americans and were altogether a queer lot. He said he didn't know much about English people but was interested in their obvious lack of sexual characteristics.[3]

DOI: 10.4324/9781003797708-16

Boehm wanted to gossip about Anna Freud and Melanie Klein, two "queens" fighting it out in the UK. Rickman gives a diplomatic response, to which Boehm barks a reply: "'Scientific differences – pshaw! It isn't that, it's a personal squabble between two women.' The degree of vehemence and attack in this conversation was most pronounced" (218).[4]

Even when Boehm tries introducing a silver lining inside Rickman's perception of him by avowing that he defied the Nazis, continuing to see Jewish patients, he gratuitously adds that "of course he could only do this if they didn't look Jewish" (219). I wonder if he thought Rickman was Jewish. Rickman:

> I had the impression that he was not telling the truth about himself when he said that he had taken risks in defying the Nazis and continuing to treat Jews, or that if this part were true, it was to deflect my attention from something else. (219)

While trying to continue with the show, even though it meant running the Jews out of town, Boehm made some awkward choices during the transition after his former boss Eitingon stepped down. He commissioned Eitingon's portrait, which the man to be honored adamantly disallowed, saw no problem asking for the return of Eitingon's personal library, which was in Jerusalem, and sent him friendly but firm reminders about money he owed for a loan from the DPG's research endowment. Schröter: "The whole episode around this loan belongs to the petty, painful dregs of the claim of continuity that the DPG alleged after 1933."[5]

Rickman's meeting with Kemper was very brief and the positive impression was largely shaped by the praise for their colleague that he heard Käthe Dräger and Marguerite Steinberg express in their respective interviews. By the dialectical twist-off that allows a style like Boehm's to be seen through, Rickman received confirmation of Kemper's exceptional status from Boehm himself, who while flunking the lie detector test dismissed Kemper.

> The conversation was in German, and he professed that he understood a little English, and when I tried him at an early stage of the interview on the simplest statements in English he professed not to understand. Later on in the interview he got excited in regard to Dr. Kemper and burst out in fluent English, "That man's a diplomat: he has no enemies and no friends." (218–219)

Strange but true: this is the bottom line of the negative assessment of Kemper's career of adaptation.[6]

While he was interviewing Käthe Dräger, Rickman got a freebie twofer when Marguerite Steinberg, who shared the flat with Dräger, joined them. This is her only sighting and there's no citing either. Like Dräger, Steinberg, Rickman reports, taught at a school that trained teachers. Both praised Kemper effusively but didn't bring up Müller-Braunschweig and Boehm (216), which Rickman interprets as a damning "no comment."[7] Could Rickman have met and meant Margarete Steinbach instead? She was adept at Romance languages, which would explain the

Marguerite. But Rickman (and Goggin & Goggin) have some explaining to do for allowing Steinbach to disappear into Steinberg.

Both Dräger and Steinbach would follow Müller-Braunschweig into the Deutsche Psychoanalytische Vereinigung (DPV), the new postwar society dedicated to Freudian psychoanalysis. When two physicians asked Müller-Braunschweig to send a training analyst to Madrid in support of the fledgling efforts of psychoanalysis in Franco's Spain, the director of the DPV encouraged Margarete Steinbach, whose Spanish was fluent and who had already lived and worked in Madrid in the 1920s, to accept the post. In 1954 she died there under mysterious circumstances. It's interesting that the Spanish request wasn't addressed to the IPA but at one remove to the director of the DPV.

With her identifying address given as Madrid, Steinbach published a long survey article, "Die Übertragung, Geschichte und Entwicklung einer Theorie" (Transference, History and Development of a Theory), which was her conscientious summary presentation of Daniel Lagache's lecture and essay "The Problem of the Transference." I looked at "Some Aspects of Transference," the lecture Lagache delivered in 1951 at the British Psychoanalytical Society, which wasn't the plenary talk given in Paris, but just the same I'm resolved to imagine that Steinbach's consummate review is a parallel effort that may well be more thorough, especially in the first part, than Lagache's own survey of theories of the transference.[8]

Like Kemper, Felix Boehm is quickly dismissed as a Nazi in the bios lite that fly around the web.[9] In Boehm's case there is the charge that he contributed to the murder of soldiers who didn't fall in line, like the malingerers and homosexuals. I don't see how such a purpose would have been in the interest of the analytic position as it was installed at the Göring Institute and its clinic. What the Nazi authorities prized in psychoanalytic psychotherapy was the practice, the practical successes, not the preaching. But in the conversation with Rickman some trigger goes to Boehm's head and colors his megalomaniacal discourse brown.

> During the war he was employed… to decide whether men were malingerers or not. If he pronounced them malingerers, they were – he drew his finger across his throat and made a noise like "esh" and chucked his thumb over his shoulder and then shrugged. (219)

It seems that Rickman may have taken this outburst to be the "something else" that Boehm was trying to hide.[10]

At the Göring Institute the analysis of the homosexuality hiding out in heterosexuality was Boehm's research specialty, which he documented in a series of articles he began publishing in 1920, numbering a series of them as his "Beiträge zur Psychologie der Homosexualität" (Contributions to the Psychology of Homosexuality). In the opening article, which bears the subtitle "Homosexuality and Polygamy,"[11] Boehm gives the fullest setting for his "contributions." The article opens in a northern city. The upper class is psychically regressed owing to a long period of political immaturity (9). Strictly protestant, the class members don't kiss prior to being officially engaged (9).

When the narrator visits a southern town it's carnival time and there are fewer fraternal organizations, no bordello, only regular hetero commitments (12). Up north, however, what follows is an innocent living out of homosexual tendencies. The schoolgirls kiss on the way home and the boys enter associations in which the mug of beer gets passed around, refilled when only half finished, then passed on to the next "brother" (10). Amorous nicknames for close friends abound. For the older youths there are bars and bordellos (the sisters hang out at the café) (9). One fraternal association selected a particular bordello for regular group visits following nights at the bar. The guys would use the same girl and share her in conversation. "The house of prostitution serves among other things the hidden satisfaction of the homosexual impulse (whereby I let stand to what degree the homosexuality is conscious)" (18). His analysis keeps turning around the homosexual component in the sexual makeup of heterosexuals: monogamy is heterosexual while polygamy is homosexual (13). In unhappy marriages both parties are homosexually disposed.

During World War One, Boehm observed that the stronger the esprit de corps among the officers, especially when facilitated by a benign friendly-fatherly attitude toward their subordinates, the stronger the polygamous tendency (15). One officer boasted that he was never the first for any girl. Disdain for the maidenhead means fleeting cum dumping in prostitutes and a predilection for adultery. For the officer to enter longer-term relations with one woman she must already be taken – and by a man he knows. Following his anthropological tour of study from the north of Germany through the ranks of the war, one of the sailors he mentioned turns out to be his patient, the first Boehm presents from his practice.

In session with this patient, Boehm touches on his coitus requirement: that he must know that another penis was inside the vagina just prior to his own entry. The patient offers a spontaneous association. "That has to do with homosexuality" (19). When Boehm touches upon this premature articulation, the patient dutifully elaborates.

> Because I am homosexually bound to my father, I seek contact in the vagina of my mother with my father's penis. This no doubt is the reason for the polygamy, I have intercourse in this way with men – an intercourse I disallow myself in any other form for moral and ethical reasons. In intercourse with a polygamous woman, I imagine contact between two penises or that the *Muttermund* [literally, mother mouth] is also a penis, that the enveloping vaginal wall is the hand holding together both penises and masturbating them. (19)

Boehm hypothesizes that cunnilingus, which is his patient's preference, elaborates the petri dish of hidden homosexual activity. "It follows from all that has been discussed so far that the vagina of the polygamous woman stimulated him because of the smell of his forerunners" (21). And by seeking out a dirty prostitute for successful coitus, the patient overcame the aversion to the dirt of the female genitalia. It's the pay dirt of intercourse with other men that he learned to appreciate.

That's why men who are homosexually inclined like to listen when women talk about their affairs (23). Getting an earful of the men boasting about their conquests also appeals to the women on this incline. Especially in couplings of two homosexually disposed polygamists, when breaking up and making up with the adulterer, the wife introduces the reconciliation intercourse with this one-time-only offer of fellatio (24). After Boehm explains the connection between homosexuality and polygamy, a female patient cries out: "Yes, but if the homosexuality is analyzed away in both parties where is the thrill of marriage? What sense does a marriage have then?" (24). That "the attempt to resolve homosexual tension through heterosexuality is something commonplace" Boehm was able to observe best during the war (24). The exemplary patient who gave Boehm so much material on the homosexual thrill side of heterosexual intercourse had a dream: "I am having coitus inside a penis that is significantly larger than mine" (25). This is to be continued, Boehm concludes, but he has already intimated this much: the dream penis is the mother's penis, the best one you never had.

In installment number II,[12] Boehm elaborates on the double penis his helpful patient from the article before presented. The patient adds a fantasy: "Mother has an elephant-size penis, but it's retracted, a horse retracts his penis, doesn't he?" (32). His greatest unconscious dread all along was that "the woman during coitus could throw out her withdrawn huge penis and hurt his smaller one or reabsorb it" (32). This leads to the challenge of getting past or in fact penetrating the woman's secret penis.

After years of identifying factory chimneys and advertising columns as phallic symbols, Boehm must modify the equation: they symbolize instead the hidden penis of the woman (33). It can surprise attack like the legendary dragon or a snake or a spider (33). "Many homosexuals experience *coitus as castration.* In this regard homosexuals with a strong narcissistic inclination imagine that the erect penis is reduced in coitus and that the woman sucks out the man's semen, going against the man's wish and damaging his property" (34). In another patient the cunnilingus he performed on his sister reflected the wish to suck out and bring to life her hidden mighty penis (34). By the homosexual dread of both acts, Boehm arrives at the parallel between cunnilingus and kissing with tongue play (34). Boehm modifies the horse phobia in Freud's case study of Little Hans. The boy's sexual research via horses uncovered the big retractable penis as a model for the penis hiding out in the mother's vagina, ready and waiting to strike. Little Hans applies his research to a plastic doll, letting a pocketknife fall from between its legs (35–36).

The third installment bears the subtitle "Homosexuality and Oedipus Complex."[13] Although a homosexual disposition is already homosexuality for Boehm, the trend he notes in not a few of his patients to see inversion as inborn, even in those who have had heterosexual experiences, seems to fulfill a fervent wish, namely, to escape the Oedipus complex. Didn't homosexual men love their mothers too much? "The most certain protection against becoming conscious of these repressed wishes is the idea that *one was born homosexual*. It is then impossible that one could ever have had sexual feelings for a female being, in other words never for one's own mother" (54). However, the emphasis on an "inverted Oedpus complex" only seeks to hide the normal Oedipus complex propping up the homosexual disposition (56).

In one analysis Boehm could even uncover that the patient's "homosexuality, that is, his male friendships, only masked his enmity toward his father and in the transference toward other men as well" (56). The homosexual acts of Boehm's patients can serve to ridicule the father while veiling the gender of the sexual object. These acts also often unman partners conceived by the patients as being on the way to sleep with their own mothers or sisters (56–57). After a long analysis a former passive homosexual, who used to get hard just seeing an officer, came to view his contact erections as potential weapons (57). Boehm adds to the compulsive striving for the male and the attendant flight from the female the wish to castrate the male partner. All the heightening of male friendship wears the mask of the normal Oedipal hate for the father (58–59). Now we can better understand the wish fantasy of releasing the father's penis inside the vagina. The homosexually disposed wants to tear it out and destroy it. This last wish is what characteristically gets repressed. Homosexuality, Boehm concludes, is the perversion in which the normal Oedipus complex has become alien to consciousness (81).

In his 1933 contribution, which was number IV, bearing the subtitle "Über zwei Typen männlicher Homosexuellen" (On Two Types of Male Homosexuals), Boehm discloses that it's the trace of heterosexual activity that makes the other penis attractive to the homosexual. Now he's talking about active homosexuality, no longer the disposition hiding out in the norm. That "in Berlin homosexual circles one says for 'masturbating someone,' 'rendering someone harmless'" (166), means keeping that subject from messing with the mother.

The ubiquity of a tendency in the hetero norm (or rather in its requisitioning in the military setting) means that homosexuality is not closeted and does not need to come out. It follows that if or when there is homosexual acting out, the outbreak can be treated within the bigger picture of heterosexuality and reabsorbed, even cured. German-language psychoanalysts had written so profusely on the meaning and treatment of homosexuality that the outside world began to wonder. Already worried about the breaking out of an epidemic of inversion, the Nazi leadership might readily have assumed that the analysts were the experts in handling this neurosis. Homosexuality and war neurosis were not so far removed, at least from the vantage of those responsible for the smoothest possible running of the war machine. Boehm, the acknowledged expert in the analysis of homosexuals, also advised on the malingerers referred to the clinic.

Boehm's unpublished "Die Bekämpfung der Homosexualität in Deutschland" (Combating Homosexuality in Germany) circulated internally in 1944 as a memo to all colleagues at the institute following an initiative to combat homosexuality and abortion. In the closing paragraph he warns against the increase (*Anwachsen*) of homosexuality as a threat to the people. Boehm sought to give guidance and, following a stricter alignment of homosexuality with criminality, still offered a way out for treatment – for example, if the patient was at the same time psychotic, alcoholic or afflicted with sleep inertia (*Schlaftrunkenheit*).

In 1950 Boehm succeeded Müller-Braunschweig as director of the DPG, which the analytic trio from the Göring Institute (Boehm, Müller-Braunschweig and Kemper) had resurrected in 1945.[14] At that time Müller-Braunschweig added a parenthesis to the organization's official title identifying its origin in the year 1910.[15] In the meantime it had become clear that Schultz-Hencke's revisionist analytic psychotherapy was the impediment in the way of the DPG's return to international psychoanalysis – certainly after Müller-Braunschweig had introduced it as the problem at the international society's first conference in Europe after the end of the war.

Müller-Braunschweig was all along planning to wield a new Freudian club to exclude the rival and his students. In other words, he was glad that Schultz-Hencke wouldn't budge because it allowed him to strike out on his own, striking two doubles in one blow. With five analysts in tow, he went to the magistrate to establish a new organization, the DPV. The founding members accompanying Müller-Braunschweig were Käthe Dräger, Ingeborg Kath, Hans March, Gerhart Scheunert and Margarete Steinbach. Several lay analysts soon followed the founding group effort to become members, including Gertrud Fuhge, Ada Müller-Braunschweig and Marie Louise Werner. It was by plan that the original group consisted of three lay analysts and three medical analysts (unlike Schultz-Hencke, Müller-Braunschweig was not a medical doctor). The symbolic constitution waited on Gerhart Scheunert, the third physician practicing analysis, who had to be cleared by his second denazifaction investigation before he could participate.

In 1951 the new organization scored international acceptance, its reward for separating itself from the continuity shot of the Göring Institute's eclecticism which Müller-Braunschweig had "demonstrated" was alive and well in the DPG. It was given license to make way for postwar German psychoanalysis to begin again in the tradition of the Psychoanalytic Institute of pre-Nazi Berlin.[16] It was as though Boehm's tearful impasse fit the crime. But who committed it? In 1958 they died in swift succession, like two Bs in a pod, Boehm in September, Müller-Braunschweig in October.

Notes

1 In *Die Reinigung der Psychoanalyse*, 38, 48, 51, 54, Regine Lockot includes evidence that, forced to choose between Boehm and Müller-Braunschweig, the analysts outside the Third Reich tended to put their trust in the former and to see in the latter someone capable of adapting to the Nazi ideology. In part this view was fueled by confidential observations offered by Eitingon and Boehm in letters sent to Anna Freud and Ernest Jones. But A. Freud's trust in Boehm ended when he demanded that the Jewish analysts who had gone into exile repay their research stipends.

2 Gerhard Maetze, "Psychoanalyse in Berlin von 1950 bis 1970," *PSYCHE. Zeitschrift für Psychoanalyse und ihre Anwendungen*, 4, 25 (April 1971), 269–286. Maetze points out that Boehm's sarcasm was relentless and although it was mixed with humor that

addition was so grim that it didn't offer relief. In interviewing the candidates applying themselves toward becoming analysts he preferred using examples from the great novels of world literature "in order to get a sense of their tragic conflicts" (272). He organized private reading evenings on weekends. Every candidate had to attend and to bring along pieces of coal in exchange as well as leave some change at the door. "Boehm liked to examine the participants meticulously or amaze them" with statements like that about the legs of his female patients. "This, then, the beginner silently reflected, must be psychosomatic medicine" (272).

3 "Report on Dr John Rickman's Visit to Berlin to Interview Psychoanalysts, 14 & 15 October 1946," Appendix in James E. Goggin and Eileen Brockman Goggin (Goggin & Goggin), *Death of a "Jewish Science": Psychoanalysis in the Third Reich* (West Lafayette: Purdue University Press, 2001), 215–222; here: 218. The subsequent page references are given in the text. Like Goggin & Goggin, Lockot doesn't correct or even indicate Rickman's mistakes. In *Die Reinigung der Psychoanalyse*, 189 n. 34, Lockot notes that she translated the material as it was first included in Pearl King's 1989 publication "Activities of British Psychoanalysts during the Second World War and the Influence of their Interdisciplinary Collaboration in the Development of Psychoanalysis in Great Britain," *International Review of Psychoanalysis*, 16, 15–32.

4 According to R. Lockot's entry on Boehm for encyclopedia.com he placed his daughters in prophylactic analysis with Melanie Klein.

5 Michael Schröter, "'Hier läuft alles zur Zufriedenheit, abgesehen von den Verlusten…' Die Deutsche Psychoanalytische Gesellschaft 1933–1936," 1120–1121.

6 In his "Bericht über die Ereignisse von 1933 bis zum Amsterdamer Kongress im August 1951" (Report on the Events from 1933 to the Amsterdam Convention in August 1951), appended in Felix Boehm, *Schriften zur Psychoanalyse* (Munich: Verlag Ölschläger, 1978), 301–310, Boehm follows his fair shake in representing Schultz-Hencke's role by giving Kemper sole credit for establishing venues in the immediate postwar period in which for the first time since 1936 a new generation could again hear authentic representations of psychoanalytic thought (306).

7 In the double interview Rickman was won over by both women, although Steinberg contributed a convenient comp for boosting his assessment of Dräger, "a person of unusual integrity of character and with fine psychological perception" (216). Just the same he waffles on the extent of Dräger's creativity (216), which may explain why Kemper alone was seen as qualified to send to Brazil. That Jones wanted to send a Berlin survivor reflects the historical landmark status of Berlin on the map of international psychoanalysis, despite the opposed historical changes that had in record time passed through its turnstile.

8 Margarete Steinbach, "Die Übertragung, Geschichte und Entwicklung einer Theorie," *PSYCHE*, 7, 4 (1953), 6–25. The text also appeared at the same time in Spanish. Steinbach refers to the 1936 conference in Marienbad as convening "the most important analysts of the German and English languages" (11). She doesn't include anyone from the Göring Institute. By now the conference is best known for Lacan's first airing of his theory of the mirror stage. In the third section of her summary article, Steinbach registers Lacan's warning against the psychologization of psychoanalysis as being more heinous in its consequences than the vantage of the natural sciences on the essence of man (22).

9 We need a third term alongside a miss and a near-miss. In 2022 the Wikipedia entry (in English) on Harald Schultz-Hencke reported that he joined with other analysts who had been excluded from the leading organizations to start the DPV. Subsequently in the wake of the infighting that ensued, he created Neo psychoanalysis.

10 For more context consider a brief report published in 1942 on the department at the Göring Institute's clinic treating criminal cases, which opened just the year before:

"Kriminalpsychologie," *Zentralblatt für Psychotherapie*, 14 (1942), 37–41. This is Marie Kalau vom Hofe's only publication as an analyst. She continued and concluded her didactic analysis with Boehm (after spending two and a half years with Sándor Rado). In the first place, as she explains the procedure, a psychotherapist specializing in criminal psychology must determine whether a case of criminality shows a will to be treated and cured (38). It isn't only the shortage of therapists for this time-consuming work that concerns her. It is imperative for the sake of the reputation of psychotherapy itself that care is taken in selecting the criminals who are suitable for treatment. It is counterproductive to "make a loud gimmicky pitch for healing every case of homosexuality, for example, only to fail miserably faced with homosexual prostitution and dilapidation or when the patient remains incorrigible, adamant in seeking protection and not the cure. Such failures are damaging not for our reputation alone but because the criminals who might benefit from treatment will no longer be referred by the relevant agencies because of the negative association" (40–41). While the refrain is that a more perfect sifting of the criminal population is required prior to referral, with focus fixed on how anchored a perpetrator is in his way of life, the fact is that, from the vantage of protecting the reputation of analytic therapy, an executed homosexual is better than an untreatable one.

11 Felix Boehm, "Beiträge zur Psychologie der Homosexualität I. Homosexualität und Polygamie," in Felix Boehm, *Schriften zur Psychoanalyse* (edited by the Deutsche Psychoanalytische Gesellschaft), 9–26. Page references are given in the text.

12 "Beiträge zur Psychologie der Homosexualität II. Ein Traum eines Homosexuellen," *Schriften zur Psychoanalyse*, 31–36. Page references are given in the text.

13 "Beiträge zur Psychologie der Homosexualität III: Homosexualität und Ödipuskomplex," *Schriften zur Psychoanalyse*, 53–65. Page references are given in the text.

14 For five years the group was the Berlin Psychoanalytic Society until the Allies in Berlin lifted the ban on "German."

15 There is disagreement between Annette Dührssen and Regina Lockot about the history of this appendix long since removed. Was it added after the DPV split or was it supplied for the new start of the DPG? Probably the latter.

16 I won't be reading Alexander Mitscherlich in this book. He had little to do with psychoanalysis in Berlin at any time. Instead, he was the impresario in Frankfurt of the return of two institutes from Nazi banishment. I touch on his season of imposture in *Nazi Psychoanalysis*, and you can read up on it in Karen Brecht's much more thorough accounts. To this day Mitscherlich is mistakenly given credit for founding the DPV. But when he did join his participation was foregrounded, a feather in the cap of the new association. Mitscherlich will return in the third book of my genealogy, which addresses the transexualism controversy between him and Medard Boss.

Chapter 13

Forays

Carl Müller-Braunschweig trained as a philosopher specializing in ethics, which he applied and explored in his first book on psychoanalysis.[1] In the summer of 1945, he wrote his second book. The new release of life after years of restrictions inspired him to compose a summary of his relationship to Freudian theory and therapy, the relationship the Nazi state had denied him. He titled the work *Streifzüge durch die Psychoanalyse* (Forays through Psychoanalysis),[2] downplaying and projecting its magnum status. In fact, the work was to be continued but he decides, in the afterword (107), to let it lie unfinished, an occasional piece like its title suggests – or the allegory of his grandiose claim to fame.

> Beginning in 1936 we were prohibited in increasing measure from representing the science of psychoanalysis in word and script… Now the time is over when we can be kept from standing up for the teachings of psychoanalysis. It's once again a cause for joy (*Freude*), it again makes sense and has a future that we now ask ourselves what our scientific position is. (7)

"There are two things that man to an extraordinary degree fears (*fürchtet*): sexual love and death" (56). Dread would have made more sense than fear, but Müller-Braunschweig's ethical view of responsibility disallows mixed feelings, really any indecisiveness or hesitation. Repression becomes an issue only when it fails.

> The act of repression miscarries mainly when a person – as is the neurotic's wont – can say neither yes nor no but only partially yes, partially no, equally recognizing and condemning an impulse. Out of this mixed attitude (*zwiespältigen Enstellung*) can be seen to emerge, inter alia, the compromise character of neurosis, the character of ambiguity of neurotic symptoms. (59)

It follows that human beings are responsible for their neuroses (60). And what else can one do but take responsibility for one's dreams as well (60)?

"I see the failure of the function of making a decision, in particular in moral matters, as one of the essential etiological conditions of neurosis" (61). That's why *Schuld* (guilt) is always a factor (61). By the failure of responsible stewardship

DOI: 10.4324/9781003797708-17

and the failure in repression that follows, impulses and stirrings pile up in the unconscious and are no longer under conscious control. The unconscious content is unfinished business filed away in such a way that it can never be found. The analogy he spins encysts the recent past, losing or flexing the unconscious content of collaboration: "it comes to represent next to the authentic and legitimate state an illegal 'state' inside the state" (62).

Depression struck after his failed attempt to turn the annexation of Austria into an opportunity for the Göring Institute to annex the Viennese psychoanalytic institute and press. The letter of reassurance he sent Anna Freud was confiscated by the Gestapo (in fact, A. Freud handed it over as evidence that she wasn't as isolated as the interrogators assumed). As a result, his public published persona came under prohibition. And yet he did continue to conduct didactic analyses under the rubric of therapy, a feint supported by Matthias Göring since his son, who had already been analyzed like the father by the Adlerian Leonhard Seif, wanted his second didactic analysis to be with Müller-Braunschweig. Like his mother he was sold on Freudian psychoanalysis. Under this quasi cover afforded by Göring's family, Müller-Braunschweig took on another didactic analysand, Ernst Schweitzer, who was Jewish. When he sent Schweitzer to London in 1939, he provided a letter of recommendation.[3]

The predominance of philosophical ethics in his thought also leads Müller-Braunschweig to overvalue the kinship between daydreaming and the night dream: "the dreamwork makes use of the means of representation of wishes and their fulfilment in order to organize an indeterminate quantity of thoughts and impulses of varying psychic character… around the wish and the content of the wish fulfilment" (42). The failed *Anschluß* and its sequelae led to his evoking a "completely other *Reich*" in his study and may explain why the excursion through psychic reality seems "at the disposal of the fantast shaping or adjusting everything according to wish and will" (66). He tarries with daydreaming at the fork in the road separating the pathways leading either to productivity or neurosis.

> The fantasying that lands in neurosis doesn't lead to productivity, which in the work of art or scientific research signifies in the final analysis a heightened interpretation and conquest of reality, but leads instead into the convent of neurosis… away from responsibility for the demands and tasks that reality sets before us. (67)

In this milieu of reality or irreality only the superego can rise above the mess of wishing to vouchsafe the non-neurotic morality of decision making.

We adapt to the external world, which results in the transformation of our organism, which "encounters the influences from the outer world by adapting to them. It adapts through differentiation. In this way the organism acquires sense organs. And so, the highly differentiated human being develops a superego" (82). The superego doesn't stem from reality contact but is the idealization of the ego. Through the superego we see reality the way it isn't yet, but the way it should be – a possible future world (82). By transforming woeful submission into subordination under one's own direction, progress is made, in Kantian terms, from heteronomy to autonomy (85–86).

Toward the end he strongly recommends the pathway trailblazed for future expeditions by Josef Meinertz's 1939 monograph, *Psychotherapie – eine Wissenschaft!* (Psychotherapy – a Science!). Müller-Braunschweig extolls the recognition therein that the import of death for understanding the perspective of neurosis embeds it all within philosophizing. Meinertz: "And even many other spiritual figures 'philosophize from death,' and not from life; thus, the archaic Greeks, Nietzsche, Klages (in particular through his flight into 'Life'), Christianity, Heidegger, probably even psychoanalysis and many more." But the relay of references reverses itself when he introduces, still on the same page, the neurotic as the potentiated caricature of the profound disposition that's able to integrate the prospect of death. "In the game the doctor plays with the patient for his soul, death participates as third."[4]

His 1927 monograph and *Streifzüge* are both well written but present rather than interpret (or interpret with) a series of basic notions of psychoanalytic theory. Müller-Braunschweig's discourse on psychoanalysis in *Streifzüge* is formally a rambling, roaming survey as though the author were holding forth while glancing at a rough draft of notes. It's the audio portion of the author photograph showing him reading *Civilization and Its Discontents*. He clearly thought the image showed him off as *Dichter Denker* but Goggin & Goggin, for example, find that what it shows is his North German peasant stock, suggesting, I gather, simplicity, even boorishness.

In *Streifzüge* he wanders through a terrain of curbed notions without saying much. In contrast, the paper he delivered in 1935 at the official anniversary celebration of the German Psychoanalytic Society is a time capsule of the international style of sexual theory, almost a parody of classical psychoanalysis. In its published version (in 1936), Müller-Braunschweig's article on penis envy and other adaptations, including lesbianism, which issue from the girl's disadvantage in the crossfire of Oedipal identifications, includes Freud's comment, in which you sense the mentor's annoyance at the narcissism of small changes amounting to nothing: "In the end the girl bemoans in your version too that she hasn't a penis for the mother, not that the mother doesn't have one for her. As is well known she believes for a long time in the penis of the mother."[5]

His Freudian article confirms that his infamous publication the year before on his discipline's worldview (a word and concept that Freud banished from the court of his science) makes a faux pitch of compatibility between psychoanalysis and National Socialism. Composed years before there was the opportunity in 1934 to publish it as feigned obeisance to the new order, it is much better reading, more concise, lively, and clear, although the message is just as limited.[6] That he senses an affinity with the book by Meinertz, with the put-on discourse of another analyst with a pronounced interest in philosophy on his shingle, need mean no more than they share the form of an elevated style. Müller-Braunschweig was Gerhart Scheunert's last didactic analyst in time for the postwar period. Scheunert, whose postwar articles we will be reading in *The Psychoanalysis of Nazism*, couldn't have had a better mentor in crafting a style that rises above its content or rather its containment of underlying hostility and self-aggrandizement. Early on, Mitscherlich commissioned Müller-Braunschweig to compose a contribution to *PSYCHE* (which, we know, he soon regretted). The long outlining presentation of psychoanalytic anthropology, the latter a topic going strong since the late 1920s in the court of philosophical influences on psychotherapy, keeps spelling out basics until one must wonder if anyone needed or wanted to read it.

The title *Streifzüge* leads in two directions; it can be translated benignly as the author's wandering reflections or with open hostility as his foraging raid. At the start of Müller-Braunschweig's 1948 study stands his controversy with Harald Schultz-Hencke, the first of the rivals demarcating the close quarters of intrigue in which his postwar struggle to restore psychoanalysis was situated. This reenactment of the alleged motivation in the years of adaptation to the constraints of the Third Reich was as posttraumatic as it was postwar. Müller-Braunschweig takes the charismatic Neo analyst with a large following (even or especially in postwar Berlin) to task for his improvement of psychoanalysis, specifically his introduction of changes to its lexicon. "One cannot foresee where one will wind up on this pathway; one concedes the words and then eventually the meaning or cause as well" (25). He's preaching to a smirking choir when he makes the understatement that the substitution of a term like "captative" for "oral" obscures rather than clarifies (25).

Müller-Braunschweig blocked the move underfoot at the Free University where he was teaching to invite Schultz-Hencke to offer seminars (seminars that would have been better attended than his own).[7] His main success in maneuvering a position for himself as a true Freudian came with the foundation of a new German psychoanalytic association, the DPV, which unlike the other, older and larger one where Schultz-Hencke figured prominently, the DPG, was then internationally authorized as psychoanalytic. The journal he started, *Die Zeitschrift für Psychoanalyse*, folded after the second issue. With how much suspicion did he recognize that the reputation of Alexander Mitscherlich was benefitting from all his own career moves that in his case fell short of fame? Müller-Braunschweig's unspoken rivalry was with Boehm, silenced by years of forced cooperation in safeguarding psychoanalysis. It must have been Boehm's idea that Müller-Braunschweig publish in 1934 the declaration of dependence extolling the compatibilities between psychoanalysis and the renewal of Germany. At the same time, it credited the author with being the duo's writer in their joint diplomatic service. As we will see in the next chapter, Rickman documented how they loudly supported one another, taking turns launching salvos in the good fight for true psychoanalysis.

Notes

1 The book with which he put out his shingle: *Das Verhältnis der Psychoanalyse zu Ethik, Religion und Seelsorge* (Schwerin: Verlag Friedrich Bahn, 1927).
2 Carl Müller-Braunschweig, *Streifzüge durch die Psychoanalyse* (Reinbek bei Hamburg: Parus Verlag, 1948), 107. Page references are given in the text.
3 Lockot, *Die Reinigung der Psychoanalyse*, 168.

4 Josef Meinertz, *Psychotherapie – eine Wissenshaft! Untersuchungen über die Wissenschaftsstruktur der Grundlagen seelischer Krankenbehandlung* (Berlin: Verlag von Julius Springer, 1939), 48. In 1949 Meinertz published a sequel in which he declared that by becoming more self-aware through depth psychology we stray into the area of philosophy in the best sense. Josef Meinertz, *Moderne Seinsprobleme in ihrer Bedeutung für die Psychologie. Ein Beitrag zur Grundlegung der Tiefenpsychologie* (Heidelberg: Verlag Lambert Schneider, 1948), 11 and 51. Another way to put it, which he does, is that depth psychology gets us out of the impasse of professional philosophers who lead a Dasein devoid of relationship. It is here that he clarifies that he's not Heideggerian. Beyond these bookends Meinertz also authored a monograph of appreciation of Wagner: *Richard Wagner und Bayreuth. Zur Psychologie des Schaffens und des Erlebens von Wagners Werken* (Berlin und Wunsiedel: Max Hesses Verlag, 1961). Perhaps because the philosophical raiment of his scientific discourse was so closely woven he could just slip it off and give like some CEO at the company dinner plot summaries unfettered by the transcription services of Oedipal profiling. It's a perfect footnote to Adorno's *The Jargon of Authenticity*. At the same time Müller-Braunschweig's reference to Meinertz is the tip of a vast undertow of Heideggerrian influence on German-language analytic psychotherapy. It took many more explicit forms than Meinertz's eclectic inclusion of it, ranging from anthropological psychotherapy to Dasein analysis. The third book in my genealogy of German psychoanalysis addresses the spread and the spreading thin of this influence.

5 Carl Müller-Braunschweig, "Die erste Objektbesetzung des Mädchens in ihrer Bedeutung für Penisneid und Weiblichkeit," *Internationale Zeitschrift für Psychoanalyse*, 22, 2 (1936), 137–176; here: 174.

6 The one over-the-top imitation-original Nazi-takeover gesture in Müller-Braunschweig's 1934 *Weltanschauung* article is the reference to "incapable weaklings" (*unfähige Weichlinge*) who become through analysis better qualified for life. But the argument or litany isn't all that unusual; the flaw, I would argue, which it shares with Neo analysis, is that it implies a fundamental view of analysis as a form of fitness training. While there's no reason why a ploy can't be continued, its status as ploy without commitment cannot so easily be argued if there was another such article by Müller-Braunschweig, which Goggin & Goggin underscore. They are referring to a 1935 text on the idea of National Socialism and psychoanalysis, which they seem to know about only from the catalogue compiled by Karen Brecht. Relying on Brecht, they write: "In that article, he had defended psychoanalysis as being consistent with the goals of National Socialism. He requested that the German government give the DPG the opportunity 'to give... our Society a specific German stamp' instead of 'the international character... with their racial differences'" (139–140). I at least can't make sense of the facsimile of a page of typescript without any reference to publication. Was it perhaps another version of the *Reichswart* article, like the memorandum that first circulated among the DPG members? Did the author of the article on *Weltanschauung* convince any party-liners back then? No surprise that when his letter to Anna Freud was intercepted in 1938, he was caught in the act of profusely identifying as a Freudian plant. That Müller-Braunschweig's article was excavated in the early 1980s and made into a scandal was less a disclosure of a secret truth and more a symptom of the repression or not seeing of the history of psychoanalysis. Goggin & Goggin were able to derive a final damning blow after talking to Lockot. Apparently, Müller-Braunschweig composed an encoded letter complying with an official request that he identify the Jewish members of the psychoanalytic community in Italy (141). Wasn't the exercise meaninglessly gratuitous – another test devised for someone under suspicion? Müller-Braunschweig did not give in to the pressure that was on him following the failed annexation to save face by joining the Nazi party.

7 Gerhard Maetze, *PSYCHE* (1971), 275. H.E. Richter describes Schultz-Hencke's seminars on the dream in terms of "Magie" and his role was that of "Zauberer." Everyone seemed hypnotized into subscribing to his views – doubles who talked and looked like him (he was always elegantly dressed). See Lockot, *Die Reinigung der Psychoanalyse*, 93.

Chapter 14

Rose

The combative style Rickman discerned in both Boehm and Müller-Braunschweig was very much in evidence at a meeting of the German Psychoanalytical Society (DPG) that five Berlin analysts and Rickman attended. Müller-Braunschweig was presiding. "He then opened a discussion on a paper by Frau Hanna Ries, a former pupil of his, who came to England in January 1939, and read a paper at the British Psychoanalytical Society on the basis of which she was admitted to full membership."[1]

> In a short time, he was denouncing the paper, thumping the table with his fist, saying it was a bad paper, it wasn't psychoanalysis, "and, just think of it, the British Society actually, on the basis of this paper, made her a member!" The theme of the badness of the paper and the stupidity of the British Society recurred during his half-hour's discourse, during which time he was several times corrected… for misquoting the paper or obviously misinterpreting it. (220)

The polemical attitude evident during the discussion was also cause for concern when Rickman attended Müller-Braunschweig's lecture, which the German analyst was supposedly pitching to an audience of uninitiated but interested students.

> Müller-Braunschweig's dogmatic and aggressive manner seemed to me to do little, if anything, to pave the way to these seminars which were the pride of the higher German educational institutions. I must say I was profoundly disappointed… Müller-Braunschweig came up to me afterwards and asked me what I thought of his lecture, whether I thought it was good or not, but I contented myself with saying that I was mainly concerned with the reaction of the audience, but he did not ask me what that was. (220)

For the record, Rickman thought Müller-Braunschweig's lecture was intellectually of such a low level that it was "far remote from the quality that you expect in a scientific man" (219).

During the discussion of the Hanna Ries paper, Müller-Braunschweig collects himself and apologizes for his display of anger, saying, however, as Rickman

DOI: 10.4324/9781003797708-18

reports, that "it was justified by his intolerance of a bad presentation of psychoanalysis" (219). Then he passes the battering to Boehm, who repeats the attacks. He, too, must be corrected when he gets muddled regarding the main theme (219). Rickman's fantasy is that in alliance with the three younger analysts he topples the doddering authoritarians.

> I proceeded to remark how strange it was that they who had only seen the paper, and some of them only in abstract, should have spent so much time in condemnation of it and have paid comparatively little heed to its clinical merits. Boehm and Müller-Braunschweig were angry, Fräulein Dräger and Steinberg agreed with me. Kemper saw the point and nodded but seemed neither to agree nor disagree.
>
> I next went on to say that the reason why she had been admitted to the Society was not on the merits or demerits of the paper – and how few people after all can write a really good scientific paper –, but on the kindness and good clinical feeling of its writer, and that we appreciated her spirit and integrity in our Society. This remark even more than the former one, produced the division which I have already mentioned, but Kemper was now warming up towards her. (221)

Regine Lockot underscores that a paper on the unwanted child by a former student forced to emigrate, a paper with which, moreover, she obtained membership in the British Psychoanalytic Society, had to be volatile.[2] This interpretation does fit the situation in which Boehm and Müller-Braunschweig were reacting against an article they hadn't read. But as Ries underscores, the title is an homage to an article by Ferenczi.[3]

Ries originally trained with Boehm, who by her own account helped her obtain the audience in London that was her ticket out of Nazi Germany. When Boehm was criticized after the war she always came to his defense. Her control analyst was Ada Müller-Braunschweig, with whom she remained good friends. I'm guessing Carl Müller-Braunschweig and Boehm were reacting against being inspected by the British Society or, rather, against the very thought that London should now be the center of psychoanalysis. Even Ries couldn't accept the recentering and liked to recall the creative spontaneity that was more in evidence at the Berlin Institute.[4] Rickman brings his share of projection to the meeting, a skewed view that Goggin & Goggin take over and install in their study with all the clerical errors and mistakes in judgment intact and uncorrected.

There's no way she gave this paper in 1939. And while it did earn her full membership in the British analytic society, it did so in 1946. Ries began seeing her patient, the unwanted child, in 1940 (153 col. 1). The young Belgian girl, Rose, nearly 18 years old at the time, requested analysis or rather its continuation. Before she fled Belgium, she was in analysis for three months. Her presenting problem was that she felt compelled to torture her family, mainly her younger sister but also her parents (153 col. 1). At the same time, she followed her mother's lead in everything, including being in analysis. She confides to Ries: "That's why I believe in her far more than in myself." Ries: "With these words Rose gave me a clue to the understanding of the phantasies… And to the uncanny power this psychotic mother exercised over her" (154 col. 1). Rose did pull up short, however, rather than follow her mother into the breakdown that, Ries suggests, rebounded enigmatically from her daughter's analysis. "When Rose's analysis had lasted for about a year, Mrs. K. had an acute psychotic outburst" and was transferred to a mental hospital (153 col. 2).

Ries seems imbued with an almost folkloric view of the psyche's powers over the physical body. It shows itself when she downplays her patient's congenital dislocation of both hips. Her mother saw the baby as dwarfish-looking and, "torn by feelings of guilt," never really welcomed the baby (153 col. 2). Baby Rose was kept in the bedroom where she was privy to primal scenes until her mother saw her looking. At that instant, in Rose's eyes, her mother turned into a witch (154 col. 1). Rose is remarkably free of shame or guilt for unconscious wishes, which makes Ries think of her as a little Eve before the expulsion from Paradise. The corresponding lack of sublimation meant, however, that at age 12 Rose left school because she couldn't absorb any more knowledge (154 col. 1).

But when Rose underwent corrective surgery, she saw the doctors as torturers, who were punishing her for her illicit wishes, castrating her, disallowing her sexual pleasure (155 col. 1). Ries links this bout of persecution mania to Rose's rejection of her mother's bias toward elevation through sacrifice (which elicits in Ries's article the only clear statement of why Rose and her family had to escape Belgium). "Rose hated the idea Mrs. K. was particularly fond of – that God wanted His chosen people to suffer much in order to increase their virtues" (155 col. 1). Rose liked to counter that God should have given his people a country for their protection. As a German Jew Ries was German, too, and flexes typical discretion when, while exhaustively listing all traumatic conditions that might have facilitated the mental disturbance in Rose's case, she doesn't even mention the Nazi threat (160 col. 1).

Rose shows improvement in the analysis; she can walk, starts seeing a boyfriend, and overcomes her chronic constipation following Ries's "casual interpretation of an anal penis" (160 col. 1). She was however not telling Ries about her sexual games with the boyfriend. "When she mentioned them to me, I advised her to wait a little before going on, until we had worked through her neurosis more thoroughly" (156 col. 1). This second "casual" interpretation or recommendation, which Rose again heeds, results in the boyfriend leaving her. In the year that follows she loses all that she gained in the analysis. "The relapse was so gradual and slow that I did not realise fully what was going on in her mind" (156 col. 1). Ries knows what she's talking about when she disagrees at the end of the article with the claim that once the transference has been established the analyst's actual personality is no longer a factor (161 col. 2). She enters her disagreement under the rubric of countertransference, which also covers her bouts of making casual suggestions.

Rose becomes increasingly apathetic – and when suicidal wishes cross her mind, she cannot fulfill them. "She bitterly accused me of having spoilt her chance of suicide since analysis had helped her to get used to her appalling state of mind and had thus diminished the courage… needed to kill herself (which I believe to be correct)" (156 col. 1–2). "I interpreted her hateful attachment as a transference of her mother relationship, stressing that hate forms a much stronger tie than love" (156 col. 2). But more than she hates Ries, Rose loathes transference interpretations. "I feel sure that Rose will only acquire a proper sense of reality when this resistance has disappeared" (156 col. 2). "She turned each of my interpretations upside down, misinterpreted my motives – in short, behaved in a clearly paranoid way, obviously imitating her mother's attitude" (158 col. 1). Rose, who is in command of several languages, gives it to Ries in her two languages: "Don't be afraid. *Geschicklichkeit ist keine Hexerei*," which Ries translates cleverness is no witchcraft (158 col. 2). In German, however, the word for cleverness or skillfulness is very close to the word for historicity.

While working through phallic material, Rose has an affair with the American friend of her best girlfriend, "another Oedipus situation" (158 col. 1). The American friend leaves and on account of the flying bombs Rose relocates to Cambridge, where she soon makes another wartime American acquaintance. That the scheduling of their sessions could be adjusted in accordance with her move makes Rose feel more independent and grown-up.

Analyst and analysand keep on going once more around the block of a borderline structure. The "censor" keeps Rose from identifying with the analyst rather than with the mother. "To my mind it depends on the eventual loosening of this grip whether or not Rose will be cured" (160 col. 2). The mother's early love for Rose was of a sexual not a tender nature (160 col. 2).

Ries sees the reality of Rose's crippled *Geschicklichkeit* and ambivalently Jewish *Geschichtlichkeit* as secondary to her psychic achievements. A movie that Ries and Rose have both seen showed psychic reality causing physical mishaps. In *The Tower of London*, a hunchback named Mord, a speaking name that in the Anglo-American audience doesn't talk to everyone, is the henchman carrying out the vocation in his name on behalf of the evil man who would be King Richard III. "This is exactly my relationship with Mummy" (159 col. 1). Each time Mord removes another successor ahead of Richard in line to the throne, the beneficiary of the "murder" knocks over another figurine in a dollhouse throne room that fills the screen. But the bleak house of Oedipus doesn't frame or contain Rose's identification with Mord. Born a monster because of "wrong intercourse" (by which she means fellatio and cunnilingus), Rose wraps her sense of self around the caged animals on screen: "I am such a cage myself and something is going up and down within me restlessly." In the primal scene, Ries recalls, Rose wanted to bite off and incorporate the father's penis. She's the cage, and the father's penis goes up and down restlessly inside it, moving like in coitus. Shared penis envy formed the "homosexual link" binding Rose to her "psychotic mother" (159 col. 2).

Reaching back through the holistic prep work for psychosomatic medicine, the old wives' tales recycling through Romantic folk literature, Ries offers a closing speculation that even a birth anomaly is not, psychically, accidental. A mother's reluctance to have a child can have an impact on the physique of the fetus.

An earlier transfer from psychoanalysis in Berlin to Brazil involved another candidate at the Psychoanalytic Institute who may well have known Hanna Ries. Adelheid Lucy Koch trained from 1929 until 1935 under Otto Fenichel and Salomea Kempner and presented her admission lecture at the meeting Jones chaired on December 4, 1935, which led to the resignation of the Jewish members. At the meeting she became through Eitingon's arrangement directly affiliated with the IPA. In 1936 she moved with her family to Sâo Paulo. The Psychoanalytic Group of Sâo Paulo, which she helped establish, was granted direct affiliation with the IPA in 1945.

Revered for her talent and skill as a psychoanalyst, she like Hanna Riess didn't publish much. When I read her 1956 article "Omnipotence and Sublimation,"[5] I wondered if her Berlin admission lecture might not have been an earlier version of the same. While the article is Kleinian, which would reflect her time in Brazil, the foundation she builds on (Freud and Ferenczi) fits her Berlin training. Sublimation, moreover, is not a key Kleinian term or concern. We begin with the foundation of her argument. If sublimation involves the transformation of object libido, as Freud advised, then sublimation relinquishes loved objects, shadow boxing between aggression toward the dead and the corollary feelings of guilt and reparation (235). All the case examples she presents in the second part of the brief article reflect mourning disorder.

Through Klein the inner spin is deepened and the Freudian equation between idealization and hidden aggression is improved upon. Idealization guarantees a good object, and this leads the child to feel omnipotent and to be capable of sublimation. It means that ultimately the idealized object can be merged with the real one. With her Kleinian glosses or glasses, Koch interprets Freud's exploration of hermaphroditism in the essay on Leonardo da Vinci as implying introjection of two good objects, one from each sex (236). If it's true that only the coupling of man and woman can overcome the incest taboo, then the requirement might be fulfilled on the inside, too. However, she concludes her discussion of the three cases by observing that "the interesting factor is that none of these patients was happy in their marriage" (237).

One patient, the youngest of many brothers, "always heard his mother remember fondly a… brother who had died at four years of age" (236). To stay clear of substitution his mother raised him like a daughter until he was of school age. He subsequently tried to be a superman and outfly gender fixity and anxiety through identification with the imaginary husband of his beloved nanny. And in his relationship to the nanny, he tried to parallel and substitute for the ideal union between his mother and her dead four-year-old. He harbored feminine and masculine sublimations and was a success socially. "He achieved true sublimations, resulting from the introjection of the good object (nanny) and the fantasy of achieving the ideal union between mother and child, hoping ultimately to restore his brother" (236).

"Another male patient, also the youngest of several brothers" suffered his terrible shock when he was four years old. An older brother got sick with TB and left for treatment at sanatoria in Europe and eventually died there. His mother became a weepy griever cut off from the living. He became a leader in his chosen field of tuberculosis research (237).

> It seems that the impulse to repair, based on infantile fantasies, gave origin to the constructive omnipotence and to the capacity for certain sublimations; but the denial of reality, which always accompanies the feeling of omnipotence, prevented the establishment of happy heterosexual relationships in real life. (237)

The female patient wanted to know who she really is. "In the transference she fell in love with me as if she were my son" (237). Her mother tired of her after two years and lost interest in daughters. Her "fantasy… was to become the ideal husband for her mother" (237).

Notes

1 Goggin & Goggin, 220. The subsequent page references are given in the text. Before his stay in Berlin on October 14–15, 1946, Rickman consulted Ries in selecting which clinicians he should interview (*Die Reinigung der Psychoanalyse*, 189).
2 Lockot, *Die Reinigung der Psychoanalyse*, 200. Goggin & Goggin chime in: "We can only assume that such a theme had to trigger very strong subconscious reactions" (165).
3 Hannah Ries, "An 'Unwelcome Child' and Her Death Instinct," *International Journal of Psychoanalysis*, 26 (1945), 153–161. Page references are given in the text.
4 She confided this in a letter to Müller-Braunschweig. *Die Reinigung der Psychoanalyse*, 200, n. 47.
5 Adelheid Lucy Koch, "Omnipotence and Sublimation," trans. Ana Pierczanski, in *The Pioneers of Psychoanalysis in South America: An Essential Guide*, ed. Nydia Lisman-Pieczarski (London and New York: Routledge, 2015), 234–238. The article appeared originally in Spanish. The English translation appeared for the first time in this collection. Page references are given in the text.

Chapter 15

Comrade Dräger

In one of the confidential asides addressed to Ernest Jones, John Rickman reports back that Kemper was for several years the analyst of the wife of Professor Göring (misidentified by Rickman as "Hermann Göring's aunt"): "he had maintained a good psychoanalytical rapport and produced good results despite the fact that he was a Communist" (217). He wasn't but Käthe Dräger was. While she didn't aspire to the profile of a published writer/thinker in psychoanalysis, in her brooding silence Dräger nevertheless drew up from her experiences during the Hitler years the best account of the so-called Göring Institute, on which subsequent histories were entirely based.[1] There are a few mistakes in judgment, as I will point out when I gloss her 1971 article (based on a lecture she gave in 1970). I will also look at her first published piece of writing, the 1946 monograph, *Praktische Psychologie als Voraussetzung der täglichen Unterrichts- und Erziehungsarbeit* (Practical Psychology as Precondition for the Daily Work of Education and Upbringing). It stems from the brief period when she thought she could identify more openly as communist after the years of her secret agency.

She really had kept silent all those years – except in the didactic analysis with Ada Müller-Braunschweig, which began in 1933. In an interview with Hans Müller-Braunschweig in 1975, Dräger claimed she was at first forthright with his mother about her own illegal political activities, but after the Edith Jacobson scandal and the restrictions that followed, she forswore her communist engagement to continue the analysis, which by all accounts was probably not the case.[2] No one knew the full extent of her involvement. Even the decision on the part of the authorities to send her to Nazi-occupied Poland to teach in 1942 could only have been based on suspicions (although her pre-Third Reich political affiliation was probably known and might well have sufficed). Because the case against her was without proof, her transfer was in lieu of punishment – and the pressing pleas (prompted by Müller-Braunschweig) that the Göring Institute made to the authorities, namely that the clinic was hurting without her, finally succeeded in bringing her back. Her transfer and return were routed through her affiliation as a teacher, which was all along her day job. Her time in Poland was her exile from psychoanalysis.

That Ingeborg Kath and Alexander Mette were communists under cover during the Third Reich is a point of agreement between interviewer Ludgar Hermanns and

DOI: 10.4324/9781003797708-19

interviewee Gerhart Scheunert in 1979. Hermanns reports a phone call with Kath in which she expressed her amazement that she and Dräger had been active communists all those years but without knowing about one another.[3] There must have been quite a few Germans who belonged to the left during the Weimar Republic who had to hide the identification during the Third Reich. In the case of Dräger, however, the involvement with and for the communist party was essential, more than an identification hidden away in a show of adjustment to the Third Reich; it was her secret life.[4] She acted as courier during the Nazi years, regularly keeping the resistance connected. However, to return to 1946, the Stalinist Eastern half of Germany and Berlin soon considered her a troublemaker, and she had to abort her attempt to integrate herself, her history, in the German communist state. By 1950 she was teaching in the West. But the result was that she again kept silent on her multitasking as teacher, analyst and political activist. No mention of her politics in the 1970/1971 history of the Göring Institute. It was a silent treatment she resolutely carried forward to and through her death in 1979: she arranged that her urn be placed in the Cemetery of the Nameless.

Asked to contribute a lecture in 1970 in her capacity as witness to the activities of the psychoanalysts in Nazi Berlin, she keeps silent in the text not only about the milieu of communist resistance in which she was so active but also about her banishment to Poland. Misled perhaps by her discretion or secrecy, Rickman had decided in his 1946 report that she was too shy to be able to make a name for herself as an analyst on the international stage (216).

Following her opening paragraph, she pronounces in the name of the audience that "we mournfully remember" the German analysts Karl Landauer and Salomea Kempner, who could not be "rescued," and John Rittmeister, executed in Berlin in 1943 (255–256).[5] In the setting of her lecture, mourning is possible. The thesis of the Mitscherlichs applies to the recalcitrant Germans at large who believe that those forced to emigrate, like her Jewish colleagues, faced a harmless fate – if not the life of Riley. "It appears to be difficult for many to imagine what it meant to emigrate under compulsion, under pressure of the immigration restrictions of various countries, and under the financial pressure of the National Socialist *Reichsfluchtsteuer* (tax for flight from the Reich)" (258). Signaling from within her *Verschwiegenheit*, her reticence, Dräger conjures the stressful situation of those critical of the regime who, staying behind in Nazi Germany, had to adapt on the outside to go unnoticed.

> To know and to have to keep silent, since talking – even talking to one's own children – signified a danger to the point of risking one's life is a major psychic impingement, which increased with the compulsion to join the war effort. Feelings of impotent anger, helpless rage, of disgust, fear and grief made major demands on the maintenance of one's psychic balance. I mention this because this psychic situation existed also for the analysts who remained in Germany, who as analysts could not be National Socialists. (259)

The stress of a double life of playacting on the outside was redoubled by the striving not to give the authorities any reason to prohibit psychoanalysis (260).

Dräger joined the Berlin Psychoanalytic Institute in 1931 and was advanced to candidacy in 1935. "We candidates and the auditors experienced the shrunken BPI back then as an oasis in the spiritual desert of the times and enjoyed a kind of catacomb-feeling of togetherness" (261). This neologizing with catacombs circulates like an encrypted slogan in the writing of the captive authors John Rittmeister and Werner Krauss and conveys the gallows humor of an inner group experience cultivated and protected by the outer adaptation of psychoanalysis to the regime. She performs her right to share this image while remaining reticent about her own political risk taking, covering it all up in the avowal that all the analysts of that time, if only by the definition of their profession, were leading double lives.

She gives 1937 as the cut-off point and recalls that in the time left before that full stop there were noteworthy seminars to attend: Müller-Braunschweig on metapsychology, Boehm on case studies and on works of literature, Kemper on Fenichel's theory of "special" neuroses (261). She gives a strong example of her abilities as an analyst in assessing Boehm's 1937 meeting with Freud in Vienna, which ended when Boehm couldn't stop talking about the hardships faced by the German analysts and Freud simply stood up and departed. Earlier Freud did say that what the Jews had always suffered the gentile analysts must now endure. "Boehm's behavior seems to me among other things the expression of the objective helplessness of the analysts remaining in Germany, whereby Boehm expected the counsel of the 'great father' without realizing that the latter was himself in great danger" (263).

The psychotherapy institute that then took the place of the BPI Dräger deems just the same a *Paradoxon* in the political situation: "Such an institute had to be full of contradictions" (263). Any focus on the individual psyche, on the inner life of a person, was opposed to the NS ideology. She must have been kept out of all negotiations with representatives of the regime if she didn't realize the authorities brought to the table the conviction that Freud's science could treat shell shock (including desertion and malingering) as well as the related disturbances of homosexual and delinquent acting out in the military setting. The inner reality of neurosis was the preamble to this successful treatment. This is where she makes the infamously incorrect statement that only 5% of the membership at the Göring Institute belonged to the Nazi party.[6] (It was more like over 30%.) Goggin & Goggin place this faux bit of math which Dräger repeats at Kemper's door.

The series of *Dreierseminare* at the new institute provided the opportunity at each meeting for a representative of one of the three main therapeutic models to take a turn demonstrating a specific model or technique. The various offers comprised a "colorful bouquet" without any system (264). The analysts drew strength from their protected and prized work at the institute's clinic. Though in time they were only a working group, their classification as Working Group A shows respect. Because key terms were used so differently, like libido and introversion á la Jung versus chez Freud, the analysts opted to offer practical presentations of in-session problems and techniques. She has positive memories of the presentations Kemper offered (264), five of which appeared after the war as articles in the *Zeitschrift für Psychoanalyse* and *PSYCHE*.

When Dräger praises Boehm's 1940 practical guidelines for the clinic as something that can still be followed today, she adds a proviso that observes the split between practice and the language of circumlocution. In the "slaves' language" Boehm had to replace psychoanalysis with "real depth-psychological treatment of longer duration" (264–265). She also cites as another instance of what could still be said at that time Rittmeister's presentation on the "tasks" of the institute, in which he argued that the therapists must set aside "the irrational sector, world view and mysticism, and avoid applying the claims of the will to a total understanding (*Allumfassendseinwollens*) of practical problems" (265).

Many *Dreierseminare* were of course led by non-analysts and Dräger at least didn't mind playing hooky. "It was possible for just a few of us to work with clinical patients at home and keep away as much as possible from the institute's events. We could do this only thanks to the protection of Kemper and Schultz-Hencke" (265). Although it was clear enough by 1927 that Schultz-Hencke, who became a member of the DPG in 1926, had his own theoretical conception of analytic psychotherapy, it wasn't until after the war that his following became the Neo-analytic group. Between 1927 and 1931 his separate piece of analytic work could be "tolerated" within "the strong group of the old DPG" (265). Dräger doesn't mention that Freud was most concerned after 1933 that Schultz-Hencke would gain the upper hand, but she does observe that "the agenda of the Göring-Institute to work out a common, generally accessible terminology suited his own agenda" (265).

Does she speak for herself when she says that although the show of resistance was always minimal in impact, and the camouflage had to be maintained for as long as one wasn't caught, psychologically the resisters could count on their self-esteem, their sense that the tyrants were neither omnipotent nor omniscient (266).

> Being a concerned opponent of National Socialism didn't make one for that reason a good analyst. But a good analyst often couldn't be interested in extramural, social, and political happenings. To combine both and engage in political resistance meant leading a double life in the Hitler era. The mortal consequence was demonstrated by the example of Dr. John Rittmeister. (266)

Because for so many of its members, the Göring Institute was a hideout, they put themselves increasingly behind a common view of the importance of psychotherapy as such. As the war escalated, afflicted soldiers were increasingly sent from the front-line hospitals to the Institute's clinic for psychotherapeutic treatment. Since military persuasion had already failed, the therapists had a relatively free hand. "How often an individual patient – paradoxically by the force of the authority of the *Reichsinstitut* – could be saved from worse scenarios could not be recorded anywhere" (266).

Kemper and Schultz-Hencke right after the war were able to consolidate the authority of psychotherapy as established at the Göring Institute in a Central Institute for Psychogenic Illnesses, "the first step in gaining recognition of neurosis as an illness at a public institution in Germany. For the first time the social insurance carriers covered the costs of psychoanalytic and other psychotherapeutic treatments" (267). The struggle that was deftly circumvented at the Göring Institute came out into the open. "It was incumbent to prove to the authorities that psychotherapy was justified and to defend analytic psychotherapy against the *Monopolansprüche* (the monopolizing agenda) of anti-analytic university psychiatry" (267).

Müller-Braunschweig overcame the deficit of Kemper's departure for Brazil and scored a double achievement when he founded a new and true German Psychoanalytic Society (the DPV) and obtained for it in 1951 recognition by the International Psychoanalytic Association. However, Dräger concludes, it amounted only to moral support for their group of nine members. But from the vantage of 1970 she knows that when Mitscherlich and company joined the DPV in the mid-1950s, psychoanalysis in Germany would again swing into upward mobility (267–268).

Before she was called on to document her experience of psychoanalysis in Nazi Berlin, Dräger's research was in the specialized area of analytic education or upbringing (*Erziehung*). In 1946 John Rickman identified Dräger and Steinberg (Steinbach!) as school counselors. Dräger's 1946 monograph is very matter of fact about the school setting, which looks to the future but is still beset by the recent past. No point getting upset at the adult culprits, like the teacher who beat the boy last year or the mother who's overworking her children to the point of incapacitating their school homework. Confrontation is pointless but one must just the same parry the blows of the years before. Undoing or containing the recent past can't succeed across the board but can only be applied to the new generation one year at a time.

> In the youths whose school years fell within the period of the Nazi regime, we can see how effective the schooling in fact was, and even where there was resistance, thinking and feeling were unconsciously influenced without their knowing it.[7]

In keeping with the agenda of the series in which her monograph appeared, which was to address general questions of education and upbringing, Dräger's coverage, which is cursory but apt, seems more a product of her time at the Göring Institute than a fresh start in psychoanalysis. But although the compass of psychodynamic eclecticism she employs shows the Adlerian approach in the ascendant, she is beholden not so much to its popularity at the Göring Institute as to Adler's and her own Marxist formation. She refers to the work of August Aichhorn (24), the specialist in psychoanalytic pedagogy who spent the Nazi years working in Vienna. At the end of her contribution, the list of fundamental studies she provides for future consultation is still a wrap with the Göring Institute.

The study is laid out like a workbook with a wide, lined margin on the right for making notes. The reader, a student training to be a teacher, wants to know about the difficult pupils he might encounter in the classroom. She starts with the pupil exhibiting a one-sided interest in one area, who in this way shows basic avoidance of emotional relationships, incapacity to connect with people, social phobia or misanthropy and, in keeping with all these motives, flight into abstraction (28). "A strong and at times one-sided interest in astronomy at the start or during puberty can mean, for example, that the pupil would like to negate his own pressing instinctual life and swerve from the earthly up to the stars" (28). After easing her reader into the main topic via a characterization sounding like folk wisdom, Dräger addresses the notion of neurotic disturbance. "The teacher must recognize where a child's behavior no longer serves his will but rather an inner compulsion. Strictness and punishment, in particular beatings, are useless, even damaging in these cases" (28). The teacher must know when to refer the neurotic pupils to a professional therapist for specialized treatment. Dräger demonstrates assessing neurosis in the case of the pupil who likes to clown around and make fun of grown-ups.

> The stunning lack of respect that's evident in the tendency to make fun of and caricature the teacher and the adult in general can at times mean more than this, it contains often already a reaction to disappointments. It can be the compensation for the overall disappointment of childlike gullibility. The small clown must find himself in a psychic situation in which he continuously needs the relief of comedy. He must, like "Punch" (*Kasper*), constantly demonstrate fearlessness, a devil may care attitude. The background to this attitude is inner anxiety… It concerns unconscious anxieties, which are completely "unreasonable," not to be influenced by understanding. (30)

In the past, children at school had to sit up straight and quiet with their hands folded and their feet placed together. This halting of all movement, including rocking back and forth, was a restraint on the arousal to masturbation. However, the stasis led to boredom and the slide into fantasy, which is a more likely masturbation resource. Masturbation poses a problem if the teacher doesn't know how to deal with it (47). While it isn't physically or psychically damaging, it can signal withdrawal of contact with the environment. If a teacher discovers same-sex mutual masturbation a big deal shouldn't be made of it, especially not in front of the class. But the teacher cannot let it go unnoticed. Undiscovered this playing around harbors the danger that sexuality will become for the children something secret, forbidden and guilt laden.

Dräger strongly objects to a notion that was still current that healthy children be kept separate from difficult ones, who should undergo instead a specialized pedagogical treatment. It is imperative that the teacher hold even disturbed children in the community (*Gemeinschaft*) because only in the community can they be properly raised (33). The teacher represents the demands of the environment and must help the children understand these requirements, to acknowledge and fulfill them (43). The teacher is authority figure and helper, leader and friend (43). "The contradiction is resolved when the teacher and the children subordinate themselves to a common task. Then there stands over the teacher here and the children there the overriding third, the communal goal, to create out of the school class a working and living community" (43). If there is a conflict in the class, the group must discuss it jointly. Even the relationship of the school children to the teacher is an appropriate topic for discussion in the group (44–45).

In her closing reflections on what the unconscious motivations might be for wanting to teach, she allows that if neurotic disturbance is present in candidates, they must be able to keep their view of the psychic structure of each pupil freed of its influence (52). But she warns against "unconscious affective reasons" like the lust for power, mastery and recognition motivating a candidate to teach. While these might have been desirable motivations in the old drill-school, they are incompatible with the new era of pedagogy. By their goodness and mildness some teachers can overcompensate for unconscious lust for power and unconscious sadism. Usually, however, "the horse's hoof" of the repressed lust for power manifests itself in activities and interventions that wield a tormenting impact upon the children (51).

Notes

1 Werner Kemper's account of the Göring Institute in *Psychotherapie in Selbstdarstellungen* is thorough and correct. For example, he says that in the final iteration of the grouping of analysts after Rittmeister's arrest and execution there was not a single Nazi. However, his admiring souvenirs of the various professionals who participated in the activities at the Göring Institute is either value-free or unrepentant. Dräger strikes the right tone in her history. I will not be addressing a somewhat earlier publication (1960s), her excellent clinical paper on *Verwahrlosung*, the German counterpart to the asocial tendency which includes, even emphasizes, squalor, because I'm saving it up for the third book in my genealogy, which reconsiders delinquency in the light of the cultural difference between the Anglo-American and the German-language approaches to the same problem. What is largely a summary of the psychoanalytic research on this problem becomes in the course of her presentation a rigorous confrontation with the recent past. She rigorously historicizes the *Verwahrlosung* symptomatized by children and teens in the 1960s as delegated by the delinquency of the fathers during the Nazi years.

2 Based on the interview with Dräger conducted by Hans Müller-Braunschweig as well as the interviews by Regine Lockot and Horst-Eberhard Richter with Dräger's close associates, Hildegard Hartung and Fred Blau, respectively, Ilka Winkelmann gives a completely thorough account of Dräger's double life. "Käthe Dräger (1900–1979): Ein Leben als Psychoanalytikerin, Pädagogin und Kommunistin," *Jahrbuch der Psychoanalyse. Beiträge zur Theorie, Praxis und Geschichte*, 55 (2007), 83–111. She discusses on pages 95–97 the likelihood that in the interview Dräger gave her didactic analyst's son the interviewee covered up that in 1935 she started covering up her political activities in the sessions.

3 Scheunert then adds that Mette too joined the communists at the end of the war out of a continuous commitment that had been kept private. Ludger M. Hermanns, "'Agieren mit weltgeschichtlichen Implikationen' Ein Interview mit Gerhart Scheunert am 21.7.1979 in Hamburg," *Luzifer-Amor*, 31, 62 (2018), 117–140; here: 124–125. However, as we will see when we devote quality time to Mette in this book's sequel, it is hard to make out more than a suspicion of his interest in Marx in the palimpsest of adjustments he was willing to make in order to keep on writing. That Mette knew Benjamin well enough to swap book reviews in the late 1920s means he was left wing. But there is no indication that he was a communist prior to joining the party after the war. And as we'll see (also in *The Psychoanalysis of Nazism*) Scheunert suffered the misprision of his false self.

4 Part of the complexity was that she sided with the other communist party that was critical of everything Stalinism came to represent. In *The Aesthetics of Resistance*, Peter Weiss gives the best rendition of this internal quarrel and its complexities, especially in the context of the shifting relations between Nazi Germany and Communist Russia.

5 That Müller-Braunschweig was able to undo the punishment of her banishment to Poland, perhaps by relegating her misguided political inclinations in the past to a neurotic condition overcome during her apprenticeship to analytic psychotherapy, might have inspired Rittmeister's confidence in his own attempts to ameliorate his sentence.

6 Was she thinking of the group of analysts rather than the membership at large? Scheunert's party membership might count as 5% of the number of analysts who were members of the Göring Institute.

7 Käthe Dräger, *Praktische Psychologie als Voraussetzung der täglichen Unterrichts- und Erziehungsarbeit* (Berlin and Leipzig: Volk und Wissen, 1946), 5. The subsequent page references are given in the text. The monograph appeared in the series *Lernen und Lehren. Methodische Schriften für Lernende Lehrer*.

Chapter 16

Child Analysis Begins in the Home of the Analyst

In the version of his report that he sent directly to Ernest Jones,[1] then president of the International Psychoanalytic Association, John Rickman adds another confidential aside, this time concerning Carl Müller-Braunschweig's family:

> His family consisted of his wife, a daughter aged about 18, who from things which were just not said I gathered had fared badly from the Russian soldiery, and a son about 18 or 19. Frau Müller-Braunschweig, an oppressed German hausfrau, listened eagerly to everything I had to say about England, and seemed to me desirous to make contact with foreigners again. (217)

No mention that Ada Müller-Braunschweig was a psychoanalyst, a colleague. The next confidential aside addressed to Jones foregrounds the "wife," who asked Rickman how German psychoanalytic colleagues would be received abroad. I guess he thought she was asking on her husband's behalf. He responds that "people of whatever nationality who had throughout trials and difficulties cherished the spirit of democracy" (218) would be welcome. He's watching out for damning non-verbal evidence in the interaction between husband and wife. "She gave a sigh of relief and looked, as I thought, in rather a frightened way at her husband. He sucked in his breath a bit, and with more hesitation looked relieved" (218). Rickman concludes that Müller-Braunschweig's personality was so "deteriorated by the Nazi regime" that he was "utterly unsuitable for employment in the G.P.R.B." (218).

A letter that has been preserved for the historical record, which Ada Müller-Braunschweig composed and sent to an acquaintance living in the United States, gives a clearer account of all that Rickman thought he could detect. It begins with her summation of the Nazi Berlin institute. "The institute under the direction of Prof. Göring was anything other than a joy (*Freude*) but also anything other than a scientific institute."[2] The setbacks in her husband's psychic well-being began with his harassment by the Gestapo because of a "harmless" letter he had sent "the daughter of Prof. Freud" (180). Depressed, then further weakened by the living conditions of total war, he fell seriously ill after the war just as he was so upbeat about being able to renew his career. She also states clearly that her daughter, like countless other young women in Berlin, was molested by Soviet Soldiers – but

DOI: 10.4324/9781003797708-20

adds that since it was a common fate, the "girls" (*Mädels*) could talk about it among themselves and thus get through and past it (181). Does she set her daughter's suffering aside so rigorously because it's overshadowed in this letter addressed to the outside world by all the German crimes against humanity?

She concludes the letter with her avowal that only now could she again feel herself to be a German. "All these years I felt ashamed to be one… We're being treated better than we expected, for, given all that Germany perpetrated in the occupied countries, things could have turned out differently for us… Germany was one big concentration camp, and we are starved for liberation and openness. But how can reparation ever be made for all the German crimes?" (181). She does, however, add that the horrific particulars in the reporting from Nuremberg are news to her and hers.

Most of the women psychoanalysts in Berlin started out specializing in child analysis. Karen Horney and Melanie Klein went on, of course, to develop theories and therapies as big as the science in which they had been schooled. But the majority remained at the starting gate, which meant that in some sense they stayed home. In her 1930 publication "Ein Fall von Schattenangst und Fragezwang" (A Case of Fear of Shadows and Compulsion to Ask Questions), Ada Müller-Braunschweig analyzed in the setting of their home her son Hans or Heini (her daughter, born a year later, is the exciting cause of his symptom picture).[3] It offers a convincing portrait of a psychoanalytic German household rendered close enough in time to the Nazi takeover that we get a sense of the continuity at stake in all the adaptations and compromises that followed.

In a different milieu, the little boy's lightly neurotic symptoms might not even have attracted any attention. But then his fear of shadows grew stronger and became phobic (134). Heini suddenly started asking questions, which was especially noticeable since he hadn't really spoken before but found and got his way non-verbally. This questioning that was his accession to speech coincided with the birth of his younger sister. His first question, the baby-talk condensation of "was ist denn das" (what is that?), is *Dattenda*? (135). It was first raised while he watched the baby girl being bathed, and he continued to ask the same question pointing to the objects in his environment as though he were going down the list of her body parts. What the sex researcher left out on that occasion, his mother points out, is her genitalia.

The questioning was as much an obstacle to his acquisition of language as its facilitator. Only when his compulsive interrogation subsides does he begin to make himself understood in regular sentences. In the meantime, his fear of shadows is in the ascendant. With a cloth he tries wiping away a shadow on the wall. Asked what he was up to, he answered, tearfully, "the shadow must go away from there" (135). That night he woke up screaming and could barely be calmed. A shadow was on the wall, and he didn't want to see it.

At this time the boy's parents had an open-bathroom-door policy, and he visited them while they were bathing. *Dattenda* met sexual difference in a guise that could not be denied, and his questioning soon became a plaint. Their household was extended family and his beloved grandmother lived with them (136). During the season of her grandson's formation of symptoms, she was very ill, which Heini did not directly experience, but which he felt, anticipated. Then she died and he continued avoiding her precincts. If the shadow is his grandmother, then it must be good, his mother suggests. If good, then he wants to touch it. Mother says OK. Can Heini touch his "little bit" (*Zipfelchen*)? He picked up this diminutive term for penis when he asked in the bathroom about his father's big one. Mother again answers in the affirmative. But then he becomes fearful and pronounces over and again the prohibition against touching the little bit even a bit (136).

Afraid of his Teddy Bear's tail, Heini tore it off and then called Teddy "dear" (137). He was beginning to distinguish between a "dear" and a "bad" shadow as well. When the point breaks off his pencil, he calls it a bad shadow. Every hole is bad. Because the drain looks mean he can't take a bath. The distinction casts a shadow on the page of his analyst mother's case study in progress: "fear of castration" (137). He looks at a photo-portrait of his father and says that his father doesn't have any hands. It must be the famous thinker-pose picture of Carl Müller-Braunschweig and his hands are prominently placed, as the parents point out to the boy. The analyst father intervenes: "Oh, you mean father has no *Zipfelchen*!" Heini laughs and slaps his father's lap, shouting "That's the *Zipfelchen*, touch it!" (137). Now "the Oedipus complex" can cast its shadow on the page (137). Heini wants to spend the night in his mother's bed. But where should your father go? He tells her that father should be put away in the attic with all the other rubbish (138).

A new series of questions arises, which can be characterized as "geographical" (138). He wants to know about different places on the map of Berlin and the means of getting there. When his parents intervene by telling him he just wanted to know where the *Zipfelchen* is, he laughs and a respite of a couple of days follows. But when the questioning returns it becomes aggressively nonsensical. A new series takes over concerning what the people (*die Leute*) will say about this or that (139). When he starts asking incessant "how" questions, his parents tell him about reproduction, and he overcomes his dread of holes. He becomes cheerful, less brooding, and begins playing for longer stretches and with increased fantasy. He learned to speak, really, to ask questions, because he needed help in figuring out the meaning of his sister's birth (143). The geographical series of "where" questions offered a repressed version of the boy's sexual research (144). What remains after the underlying conflict has been overcome can be greeted as sublimation. The series of questions about what the people say hails from a higher office than that of his father. While his analytic parents are tolerant, "the people" are not happy about his destructive wishes.

Ada Müller-Braunschweig knew her future husband for quite some time before he proposed marriage – he was her training analyst and colleague at the institute. His first wife couldn't have children, and he desperately wanted a family scene. But he respected his first wife, claiming that he had learned from her that women fully had the right to develop as individuals. He never removed her portrait from his study wall.[4] The second wife accepted the proposal and fulfilled her reproductive part in their arrangement. Taking a break from her career, she studied and took notes on the scene, making it the scene of her writing about it.

Rickman wasn't alone in seeing that the introspective Ada was oppressed by her husband. To which we should add, since Rickman wasn't cognizant of her status as analyst, that her analytic development was probably stymied as well by working in his "shadow."[5] She might otherwise have published more than she did, indeed, more than he did. The 1930 article wrapped around the transcript of what she observed is far more analytic and disambiguated than her husband's published work. But his death wasn't the door shutting so there could be another door opening. When she did survive him it's not like she started to thrive or begin anew, but in the two-year span of mourning died, too.

In the mother's article analyzing her young son, she claims at one point not to have understood Heini's question, even allowing that she perhaps didn't want to understand it. He asks what would happen if he remained on the tracks while the train in which his mother and father were traveling was approaching. She answers that he would be run down. That is the right answer. But Heini was manipulating them to share his fantasy of participating in the parental coitus (145). He had already asked his father the same question and Carl answered that of course he would invite Heini to join them in the train so he wouldn't be in danger. When his father explained that the baby can't come out of the *Zipfelchen* but must emerge from the mother's hole, Heini recognized that woman was like a candy machine: you drop in some change and cream bonbons drop out below (141).

Ada Müller-Braunschweig saw that the projective casting of a shadow outlined the rise of an erection (142). If the father's penis could be a *Zipfelchen*, then the tumescence of Heini's little bit can count as a member of the cast. The bathroom scene ended up upsetting the boy so much that the parents decided henceforth not to leave the door open for his research – and the author, on second thought, even wonders whether the open-door policy was ever a good idea to begin with (136).

Hans Müller-Braunschweig spent many years integrating his artistic interests within his decision to become a psychoanalyst, opting for a mode of treatment he eclecticized as body-based therapy. His mother could be seen to model this integration process. I'm thinking of the moment in the article about her son's passing phobia when she touches on the problem of mourning. By combining the masturbatory significance of the shadow with his grandmother's death, she recognized that her little boy had encountered "the proof that something dear could disappear" (142–143). Heini became an analyst after both his parents had passed.

In 1983 his dead father's article "Psychoanalyse und Weltanschauung" surfaced, was reprinted and discussed in the journals of his field. In his contribution the son denies that there was a Nazi commitment in his father to match the faux enthusiasm of an article tweaked to sell the cause of psychoanalysis to the authorities.[6] Was the article known to his psychoanalytic colleagues, even at the time, appearing as it did in a Nazi newspaper?[7]

Notes

1 The official report was submitted to Sylvia Payne, then president of the British Psychoanalytical Society. Why he sent a more confidential version to Jones no doubt reflects their longer standing association as well as Jones's greater familiarity with the persons interviewed.

2 Cited in Christiane Ludwig-Körner, *Wiederentdeckt – Psychoanalytikerinnen in Berlin* (Gießen: Psychosozial-Verlag, 1999), 180. Ludwig-Körner's source is Regine Lockot, *Die Reinigung der Psychoanalyse* (1994). Subsequent page references to the letter in Ludwig-Körner are given in the text.

3 Ada Müller-Braunschweig, "Ein Fall von Schattenangst und Fragezwang (bei einem dreijährigen Knaben)," *Zeitschrift für psychoanalytische Pädagogik*, IV, 4/5 (April–May 1930), 134–145. Page references are given in the text.

4 See Ludwig-Körner, 176.

5 As in the title of one section of the entry on her in Ludwig-Körner, 177.

6 Hans Müller-Braunschweig, "Fünfzig Jahre danach," *Psychoanalyse und Nationalsozialismus. Beiträge zur Bearbeitung eines unbewältigten Traumas*, ed. Hans-Martin Lohmann (Frankfurt a/M: Fischer Taschenbuch Verlag, 1984), 113–119. The 1984 volume collects the most important essays responding to the growing debate on the history of analysis at the Göring Institute.

7 In Helmut Dahmer's response to the reprinted Müller-Braunschweig article in *Psychoanalyse und Nationalsozialismus*, we learn that Wilhelm Reich, who was watching Nazi publications from his place of exile, discovered the Müller-Braunschweig anomaly in a Nazi paper. He reprinted it for the first time in the premier issue of the journal he founded in Copenhagen. Otherwise, since it was only available to Nazi activists who liked reading their own propaganda, it might never have been uncovered.

Chapter 17

Fitness Regimens

Because the author formed a triangle with Kemper and Rittmeister at the time of the latter's arrest and imprisonment, we already consulted Harald Schultz-Hencke's study *The Inhibited Man*, the focus of their three-way engagement. I argued that the two survivors of Rittmeister's execution who were, finally, closest to him at that time joined forces after the war in laying the groundwork for restarting analytic psychotherapy, a plan compatible with Schultz-Hencke's fundamental views and, confusingly enough, with the layout of therapeutic eclecticism that was the hallmark of the Göring Institute. But their success story concluded for Kemper upon his departure for Brazil, the onset as well of his re-Freudianization. While Kemper's role of founding father of official psychoanalysis in Brazil went back to the future, Schultz-Hencke proceeded to make his longstanding revisionism official by coming out as a Neo psychoanalyst. That they remained good friends in the years that followed points to the real basis for their cooperation in the immediate postwar period.

Harald Schultz-Hencke was a bona fide psychoanalyst but was committed already during the Weimar period to revising the terminology of Freud's science. While he was exceedingly influential at the Göring Institute, he was kept from a leadership position at the Göring Institute because he had a Jewish ex-wife. The changes he proposed already in the 1920s, which anticipated the program of synthesis at the Göring Institute, would have made him the poster boy of Nazi German psychotherapy if he had in fact been a political opportunist, which he was not.

No doubt following the prompts of Ernest Jones, John Rickman did not meet with Schultz-Hencke during his 1946 on-site visit assessing what remained of psychoanalysis in Berlin. But by leaving out an analyst who was by all accounts one of the leading clinicians at the Institute, his appraisal lacks context, continuity and history. We will read closely Schultz-Hencke's text on fitness because it raises the question of how Nazi the content is (even as we note the continuity of its perspective going back to the late 1920s and looking forward to a new postwar consensus). "Fitness" is almost the abstract and advert of the *The Inhibited Man*, Rittmeister's inspiration, as we saw, for his neurosis defense.

In 2003 Zvi Lothane makes a shift in his assessment of the two "Nazi" articles in defense of psychoanalysis penned by Müller-Braunschweig and Schultz-Hencke.[1]

DOI: 10.4324/9781003797708-21

He does the research and discovers that Müller-Braunschweig's article in 1934 was the second or third version of a lecture he first gave in 1929 at a psychoanalytic conference, then published in 1930 in a journal for psychoanalytic pedagogy. It was reprinted in 1931 in the *Almanach der Psychoanalyse*. The only thing added for its 1933 publication is the buzz line: "Psychoanalysis works to remodel incapable weaklings into people who can cope with life (*lebenstüchtigen Menschen*)." Lothane points out that the German word translated as "weaklings," *Weichlinge* not *Schwächlinge*, should be better translated as "mollycoddles."[2] While he mentions before closing that according to Nitschke leniency was beginning to be shown Schultz-Hencke in the historiography of German analysis after 1933, Lothane himself views the man, although his first wife was Jewish and he was steadfast about not joining the Nazis, as integrating his work into the new regime. That advocates for a hard but fair assessment of Schultz-Hencke's article "Tüchtigkeit" (Fitness), which appeared in 1934.

Müller-Braunschweig added a sentence to an old article on the ideology or worldview of psychoanalysis and published the result in a party paper for a Nazi readership. That he didn't even go to the trouble of composing a new article in the light of the takeover reinforces the superficiality of his feint. Schultz-Hencke's fitness program by contrast is a concise presentation of his overall revision of psychoanalysis since 1927. That it is styling like a Nazi approach to hailing, I mean healing, is, ironically, a historical accident, one that he however augments at times to the point of parody.

Was he joining Müller-Braunschweig in his capacity as one of the three figureheads of the truncated analytic group in the charade of soul mating? Does he affirm elsewhere in his work that the will, blood and life are determining values in psychotherapy? He does, but only in this article can he be considered strident.[3] I would wager that he let all his negative transference hang out in this comicstripped-down polemic, in which he advocated – in the name of the common sense of the people – his vision of a less speculative, less controversial version of Freud's science. That he here, too, gives it the name of his own, Desmolyse, is almost charmingly clueless. For the rest, however, he shows an impresario's media savvy, punctuating his short article with section titles that are like pull-quotes. Was it because of this performance – tipping the scales that fall from the eyes of insiders – that Schultz-Hencke's colleagues were inclined to assume that all his work published during the Third Reich was in code, even *The Inhibited Man*, so that the still psychoanalysis-syntonic message was transmitting between the lines?[4] That *The Inhibited Man* could be received by fellow analysts at the Göring Institute as a coded innovation of and within Freud's science shows that the translation problem in which Schultz-Hencke was engaged since the 1920s came to syndicate the overall crisis of adaptation facing all the analysts after 1933.

On the page of this academic journal Schultz-Hencke lays out his argument like a newspaper article, the actual status of Müller-Braunschweig's contribution. One wonders if both articles were at first composed with a non-specialist, non-academic readership in mind. The mission Schultz-Hencke chose to accept with "Tüchtigkeit" was to make a pitch for psychoanalysis, still the discipline to which he was assigned, in a special Freud-bashing issue featuring the leading Adlerians and Jungians (and Jung himself) but only the one psychoanalyst.

Schultz-Hencke begins in the practical register.[5] What he has going for him in this inimical in-crowd is that the analysts were, by all accounts, the proven clinicians who got results. In accord with the hit list (the will, blood, and the life), Schultz-Hencke proclaims psychotherapy's goals and worldviews to be those of the people (85). This introduces his choice of the key term of his polemic, *Tüchtigkeit*, which is hard to translate. Lothane wonderfully offers "fitness," which I am using, but the German word denotes rather efficiency, prowess and hard work. It is in the first place, Schultz-Hencke writes, the power (*Kraft*) alotted human beings, the "pound" they must manage and maintain (*verwalten*) (85).

The individual with a healthy pensum of power and strength doesn't just go his own way. Instead, he is duty bound to serve the community in which he lives. It goes without saying that wherever the individual can help he gives a hand. No one lacks the talent for pitching in.

> Not because he is driven to do so, to forgo his own pleasure and make a tiresome sacrifice, but to live truly and become who he is he must place his abilities at the disposal of something greater than himself. (85)

But: he must have his collected power available to apply it in this way.

The neurotic doesn't have all his expansive powers in a row, at least not to the extent that his "total nature" should allow (86). For, he has lost a good deal of his expansive power to his symptomatology. This power must and can be restored to the individual and thus to the community. But is every neurosis structured in this way? "Here differentiating science applies and sets limits" (86).

Symptoms can be loud or slight, but heavy-duty symptomatology may be easier to lift than symptoms lite, which are the difficult ones. Recognition of this fact has not penetrated the scientific world although it is essential to the work of assessment. Neurosis weighs in heavy or lightweight. A light neurosis, often the consequence of some traumatic event falling into an active life, can abate spontaneously – in half a year, a year, a year and a half. The manner of therapy suited in this case is incidental. Even occupational therapy can give support. Here eclecticism is as justified as it is inevitable. But the treatment is in each case causal not symptomatic. Schultz-Hencke is masterfully inculcating his readership with the paranoia of increments of taking a pervasive illness seriously – the milieu of the psychotherapy of everyday life – so that he can set forth the importance of choosing the right therapy for treating true neurotic illness. The fitness of the neurotic must either be restored or constructed, which is the basic but profound difference between light and heavy cases. It marks the place for the existing opposition among the psychotherapeutic schools and explains the resoluteness and self-certainty with which they ply their convictions.

For the treatment of heavy-duty neurosis Schultz-Hencke pitches colleague J.H. Schultz's autogenic training. Schultz also contributed to this special issue. His article is an assessment of the Eastern therapeutic practice of yoga and not an evaluation of the limits of psychoanalysis. If Schultz-Hencke was an outsider by dint of his longstanding wish to reform the language of Freud's science, Schultz was not an analyst but a medical psychologist whose non-partisan view that psychoanalysis, as the most advanced psychotherapy, must play a central role in unifying all depth-psychological treatments made him an ally of the analytic group. Because his ex-wife was Jewish, he could not hold a directorial position. Schultz-Hencke, the other leading figure, was, as noted before, also kept from a directorship by his ex-wife being Jewish. A history of intermarriage also meant you couldn't join the Nazi party, which didn't even cross Schultz-Hencke's mind. But judging by photos portraying him at this time J.H. Schultz might well have been restrained by his ex-marriage from what he really wanted, a more complete adaptation to the status quo through party membership.

Autogenic training, Schultz-Hencke argues, can go far toward introducing a new order for the personality. Here the possibility of choice opens wide between deeply organizing self-inspection and other methods. Integration in the great world of human confrontation with life and with one's own interiority is one way to go. Starting out from the dream, and including its syndications in cult, ritual, legend, saga and religious doctrine, is another approach that can give order to the individual life. Though not identified in the article this seems to cover Jungian analysis. But Schultz-Hencke wonders whether applications of the psychology of the *Volk* can extend to the heavyweight neurotic conditions.

It is no longer the time for assessing the efficacy of existing methods. We must only classify how far a method of treatment reaches into the realm of neurosis and what magnitude of inhibited forces of expansion can they counter and reverse – in sum, to what extent can they turn unfitness into fitness. Finally, which method can discipline the new fully unfolding expansion powers without exchanging them for a new inhibitedness. Only then can we recognize the benefits of "the heavy artillery fire" (*das schwere Geschütz*) of individual psychology and psychoanalysis.

Following his brief representation of the other German psychotherapies available for the treatment of neurosis, light or heavy, Schultz-Hencke pitches psychoanalysis as a match for the inhibited condition. If only to echo the special issue, he must first banish the "orthodox" adherents lest the verifiable basis of psychoanalysis itself elude his readership. Freud is named while assessing the damage of his second thoughts. Psychoanalysis is not a new psychology but an excerpt from psychology. It's not man as such that it addresses but the inhibited man, man held back from engaging his own expansive powers. Cleansed of the gratuitous speculations and theorizations that are in truth wildly uninhibited, psychoanalysis stands on its solid basics. It is the doctrine of the inhibited Everyman.

In example-rich pages Schultz-Hencke evokes the milieu of what would be housed at the Göring Institute as an insider involved in its foundation from the start.[6] He either sees the future or provides the model for what would be possible there and then. The sexual or libido theory only gets in the way of the fitness of psychoanalysis for the task of restoring the expansive forces.[7] To view the treatment of the homosexual neurotic as the patient's conversion to heterosexuality reflects the bias of the theory (94). Instead, the neurotic should be turned into a proper man or proper woman, a reformulation that reflects a difference the scientific community keeps on ignoring between a real man and just another heterosexual. A proper man is no doubt straight but to stop there limits the prospect of full controlled release of his expansive forces (94).

Uninhibited psychoanalysis has pursued three themes that have nothing to do with science or therapy: the criminal didn't do it; religion stems from the Oedipus complex; there is a special psychoanalytic pedagogy (96). The truth is that many criminals are neurotic, and that the psychologist can offer valuable assessments of the criminal as a neurotic. But it is up to the judge to determine the verdict. It is over the top to characterize religion as infantile. But there are worshippers who are inhibited and must be treated as neurotics (and not as religious practitioners) (96). Anyone who has dealt with the developmental history of the inhibited knows something about moments in the education and upbringing of children that produce inhibitions or contribute to their later formation (97). This knowledge belongs to a psychological and not a philosophical pedagogy. Again, psychoanalysis as an "aspect of an aspect" is not able to subsume and renew pedagogy. A larger claim only compromises the scientific standing of psychoanalysis. If you're going to wear your glasses, to use them, you must keep them clean. Schultz-Hencke has knocked out the speculative excesses of the Freudian school so that psychoanalysis (and the readership of his article) can see better what can be done.

At the first conference after the war where the German contingent was welcomed back, it was without any warning that Müller-Braunschweig delivered immediately following Schultz-Hencke's lecture a methodical critique of his colleague's revisionism, one that the international audience could applaud. His critique of Schultz-Hencke's lecture became the celebrated cause of delivering West German psychoanalysis from the influence of the Nazi years.

Jones was of course privy to Freud's early suspicions of the man and his proposed changes to the terminology, but by opting to dismiss Schultz-Hencke's presentation as impossible to follow through the thicket of the clinician's private narcissism of words he was wrapping a colleague's Neo, like that of Wilhelm Reich before him, in the impasse of psychotic transference.

The setting of distrust and distancing toward the German colleagues, which benefitted Müller-Braunschweig, only alienated Baumeyer, Boehm and Riemann, who sided with Schultz-Hencke in the conference showdown. Riemann went so far as to propose that the German group quit the international association. After all they had suffered during the Third Reich on account of their commitment (*Einsatz*) to psychoanalysis Riemann found the attitude of the leadership of the IPA uncollegial, evidence of a tendentious resentment from which the international colleagues would perhaps never free themselves. Why should Schultz-Hencke resign? To facilitate the DPG's alleged prospects for international recognition? What convenience story was it this time that should motivate an esteemed colleague to withdraw voluntarily from the organization to which he belonged? In a letter to Müller-Braunschweig, Kemper, while admitting that Schultz-Hencke's emphatic correction of Freud was a performance that rubbed the wrong way, protested that there were far greater divergences from Freudian doctrine in international psychoanalysis than in their colleague's proposals.[8]

Notes

1 In "The Deal with the Devil to 'Save' Psychoanalysis in Germany," *The Psychoanalytic Review*, 88, 2 (2001), 195–224: here: 202, Lothane accessorizes Müller-Braunschweig like Felix Boehm "with proven Nazi affiliations and connections."

2 Zvi Lothane, "Power Politics and Psychoanalysis – An Introduction," *International Forum of Psychoanalysis*, 12, 2–3 (2003), 85–97. This was a special issue on "Psychoanalysis and the Third Reich" that Lothane guest edited. I consulted the version on researchgate.net, 1–16; here: 10–13. Oddly, Michael Schröter offered an alternate origin story for the *Weltanschauung* article, which comes down to the same mitigating contextualization (although Schröter emphasizes that Müller-Braunschweig was of a Christian anti-left persuasion). Schröter tracks instead a memorandum Müller Braunschweig composed in 1933 which was at first his and Boehm's secret but then circulated among the members of the German Psychoanalytic Society (DPG). While many took offense, others found the show of indignation laughable. Schröter quotes Fenichel's comment in the *Rundbriefe*: "If one for existential reasons composes a memorandum addressed to a particular office and with definite goals in mind, then the adaptation-style is necessary and at most a bit of fun entertainment (*Gaudium*) but not a desecration of the cause." Again, the truly objectionable sentence was added to the article as it was published in the Nazi paper. See Michael Schröter, "'Hier läuft alles zur Zufriedenheit, abgesehen von den Verlusten…,'" 1099–1102. In composing the memorandum, for example, Müller-Braunschweig may well have recycled the earlier article(s) that Lothane discovered. That the article(s) can be seen to encircle a point of fixation in Müller-Braunschweig's thought and writing is another story.

3 Harald Schultz-Hencke, "Die Tüchtigkeit als psychotherapeutisches Ziel," *Zentralblatt für Psychotherapie*, 7 (1934), 84–97; here: 85. The subsequent page references are given in the text.

4 Gerhart Scheunert says as much on behalf of the analytic group back then. See the 1979 interview Ludger M. Hermanns conducted with Scheunert in *Luzifer-Amor. Zeitschrift zur Geschichte der Psychoanalyse*, 31, 62 (2018), 117–140. His recollection of what they thought Schultz-Hencke was up to is on p. 123.

5 According to Schröter (1108), the Nazi government immediately gave psychoanalysts affiliated with the Berlin Psychoanalytic Institute's clinic permission to (continue to) treat. The permission to teach, however, wasn't granted until 1936.

6 Of course, Göring and Schultz-Hencke worked closely together but the question remains whether Göring did anything on his own or was he mainly a figurehead motivated and propelled to perform his acts of founding and leading. In name, Göring was the founder in 1933 of the Deutsche allgemeine ärztliche Gesellschaft für Psychotherapie (German General Medical Society for Psychotherapy), which can be seen as the staging ground for the later institute. And he already placed Schultz-Hencke on the society's Board as the representative of psychoanalysis. It was arguably in this capacity that Schultz-Hencke wrote the fitness article. See Schröter, 1103–1104. What ensued – lasting even through the early postwar years – was the farcical feuding between Müller-Braunschweig and

Schultz-Hencke. I read in Zvi Lothane's "The Deal with the Devil to 'Save' Psychoanalysis in Germany" (220) that Schultz-Hencke voted for Eitingon in the first election that rationalized adaptation to the new regime's anti-Semitism laws – but that also means he voted against Müller-Braunschweig. Schröter (1105) counts two proposals for the constitution of the new institute submitted to Göring by Müller-Braunschweig and by F. Künkel in 1934. Müller-Braunschweig's proposal was already invested in marginalizing Schultz-Hencke. However, the puppeteer's fitness article comes closest to what was pursued in Göring's name.

7 An expurgated version of the article, which lacks these three or so pages, is in the foreground of Internet searches. It was scanned from Wolfgang Bock's 2018 study *Dialektische Psychologie: Adornos Rezeption der Psychoanalyse*, in which it is one in a relay of appendices comprising the *Nachwort*. Among Bock's appendices are many hard-to-find articles (by Adorno and Marcuse, for example) and I was grateful for the easy access. However, I had read the Schultz-Hencke article before and taken extensive notes, which led to my discovery of the missing pages. In the opening pages of *Dialektische Psychologie* the author's name is awarded a place: Rio de Janeiro. This fully manifests on virtually infinite pages the legacy of not-see psychoanalysis. See Bock's "Resümierendes Nachwort:" https://searchworks-lb.stanford.edu.

8 When he was back in Berlin in 1967, Kemper was invited to give a lecture at the Berlin Psychoanalytic Institute that the DPV had reestablished. The protocols whereby he was asked to prove his allegiance reminded him of being back in the Third Reich. Only because of the continuity that he and Schultz-Hencke had provided through the *Zentralinstitut* could the analysts today (in other words, under less dangerous conditions) allow themselves the luxury of exclusively carrying out the differences between analytic approaches to the point of dividing their own house. See Regine Lockot, *Die Reinigung der Psychoanalyse*, 177, 223–224, 231, 219–220, 220, 261–263.

Part Four

The Author of JR's Demise

Chapter 18

Whose Language Was It?

Not convinced by the detective work of my predecessors, who claimed to find through the transferential history of the training analyses passing through the Lobo scandal a reopening of the Rittmeister cold case that nails Kemper as the Nazi informant, at the end of the row of chapters investigating Rittmeister's analytic and therapeutic colleagues we are left with the non-analyst Werner Krauss. A scholar and author of fiction, he was Rittmeister's closest friend at the time he, too, joined the resistance and was arrested and imprisoned but not executed. They were captive authors in their separate cells trying to assemble a case for a more lenient view of their treason.[1] Both were, after all, of good stock and their political activities could be seen as symptomatic of neurosis and, since the condition was treatable, they could be brought back home into the Reich. The network of petitioning to make the case began with the prison writing of both men, an open book secretly addressed to the examining authorities. Rittmeister failed to overturn the death sentence while Krauss succeeded in ameliorating his own sentencing into a five-year prison term. Does the divergence in their destinies go beyond Rittmeister's prominence, which was just asking for a lesson to be made? He was, after all, the director of the clinic at the research institute ranked essential for the war effort.

Rittmeister had to fail in his efforts to influence the verdict because it was too late for leniency. The gambit of the recovered neurotic had been overplayed. Harro Schulze-Boysen, the leading figure of the *Rote Kapelle*, used his high-ranking position in the Air Ministry to obtain for Soviet intelligence advance information that helped stop the German momentum. In 1933 Schulze-Boysen had already been arrested and imprisoned for a show of political resistance. He knew how to style his recovery from neurotic influence, heralding his full return to Aryan stock worthy of a prominent position. The homoerotic investment in a hero reclaimed for Nazi Germany was interpersonally active in Hermann Göring's friendship and protection. That in 1933 Schulze-Boysen was forced to witness the execution of his Jewish friend and compatriot belongs to stock footage of German homoerotic history, reprising Frederick the Great's captive audience under his father's direction at the execution of his best friend with benefits. Hermann was raging over his seduction by the good-looking deceiver and traitor, and Schulze-Boysen was strung up to die, an insult since by his rank it was his right to be decapitated instead.

DOI: 10.4324/9781003797708-23

While his team of supporters was documenting the case of the absent-minded academic recruited by individuals better suited for political involvement than he could ever be, Krauss obtained permission to work on a scholarly study in his jail cell. Under the cover of that project, he also secretly wrote his novel *PLN*, a satire fictionalizing Krauss as the postal minister of Halyconia, the fictionalized Third Reich, and Rittmeister as the psychiatrist who recruits him for the fictionalized resistance group. Whether it's the teen's diary or a prison novel, there is no secret writing, and the illusory confidentiality will be breached, and the secret communicated.

The book that encrypts Krauss and Rittmeister's sojourn in the *Rote Kapelle* in Nazi Berlin is at the same time a language satire that explores the mystery of an official discourse that operates as a correctional institution but must at the same time fashion an Ersatz language out of the stores of literal, etymologically transparent words characteristic of the German language. While the official discourse of *Blut und Boden* was the address of the middlebrowbeat of talking heads, the bulk rate of Nazi language was allied to and vied with the talk that walked the streets of Berlin before marching down the ranks of total mobilization.

The language Krauss fictionalized in his prison novel while composing in elevated academic German his study of Gracián he theorized in an article published right after the war. But he found himself doubled and denied when Victor Klemperer put out his shingle right next door not only as a scholar of Romance languages and literatures, but also as the author of a study of the language of Nazi Germany. One is tempted to think that this study really had to win acclaim, which it did, because there was no other on this topic – if it weren't for Krauss's work standing by, overshadowed by the doubling. The difference between them was that Krauss recognized the role of adolescent idioms in the constitution and maintenance of the language.

That the doubling between the two East German academics enfolded the missing link of adolescence is weirdly confirmed by stations in the dramaturgy of the members of the Klemperer clan starting over in California. Before returning to Western Europe and countering his cousin Victor's postwar identification as a citizen of communist East Germany by becoming a citizen of Israel, Otto Klemperer was the conductor who put the Los Angeles Philharmonic on the map from 1933 until 1939. That was enough time for his son to catch the acting bug. Victor's second cousin, then, was Werner Klemperer, who started appearing on small and big screens in the mid-1950s and ended up best known for his role as Colonel Klink in *Hogan's Heroes*.

The 1947 study of the language of National Socialism, *LTI – Notebook of a Philologist*, folds out of the extensive diaries he kept during his stint in the Third Reich as Jewish husband of an Aryan wife.[2] Although the couple was regularly harassed and berated by the Gestapo, as long as the wife stood by her man he was safe, until, that is, a closing clean-up at the end of the war almost claimed him – on the eve of the fire-bombing of Dresden, which allowed the couple to survive the regime on the leveled playing field. Which only goes to show that even Allied overkill was justified against the criminal state. The focus of *LTI*, then, with its journaling provenance, is on Klemperer's experience of a lingo that infiltrated his place of work overnight, and which he subsequently observed at the distance and through the filtering of his shunned status.

In 1944, for example, he gets hold of a newspaper and reads in the author's press release a sampling of a new study by Dr. von Werder on the "psychic reality" of rural migration. It is an example of the Nazi "Tiefenstil" (depth style) that was cultivated in no time in every academic discipline.[3] The predilection for German-only neo-archaisms notwithstanding, Klemperer argues that it's not a folksy discourse but seems designed rather *not* to be readily understood by the people. Klemperer underscores instead the salient feature of the language at large, the alternation that Goebbels mastered in his tirades, the back and forth between, as Klemperer puts it, hot and cold showers – the jumpy switching "from a learned tone to a proletarian one, from sobriety to the tone of the preacher, from icy rationalism to the sentimentality of a manfully repressed tear" (238).[4] Goebbels, in other words, was fluent in the faux profundity of the ideology but at the same time commanded all the other registers of the loud organ concert of Nazi-speak.

Goebbels claimed to read his speeches from the lips of the people, and was fondly known as "the Doctor," awarding him an aura of healing and *Heil*-ing, although his degree was in German literature. By sliding "from Fontane's simplicity and Berlin gruffness to the pathos of the evangelist and prophet," the Doctor's output constantly attracts and rebuffs, Klemperer advises, leaving no time for critical reasoning (238). This fits a bit of national character psychologizing on Klemperer's part: "alongside the craving to dominate the world was a desire to escape it" (246–247). Klemperer enters this mindset when he avows the fundamentally Romantic quality of the Teutonic character: the feeling that propels you towards the infinite (246). This reaching out allows symbolic speculation to encroach on *Wissenschaft*, a term we tend to translate as science, which in English is short for natural science. But *Wissenschaft* is also used in German to designate academic scholarship in the humanities. Klemperer does mean natural science, however, when he writes: "The construction of the Aryan has its roots in philology rather than science" (130).

Klemperer identifies the milieu of literary freedom in the Weimar Republic as the precondition for the development of Nazi-speak.

> The result of all this was not only that there was a wholesale blossoming of the principal areas of language – encompassing spoken, written, journalistic, academic and literary forms – not only that the widespread literary currents… could prosper, but also that in all disciplines entirely individual linguistic styles could evolve. (19)

Nazi lingo, though unfree, follows rather than contradicts this *Aufbruch*, a new start and departure (19).

What was celebrated as profound was also limited. But that's also the limit imposed on its analysis. Early in the study Klemperer summarizes the metabolic process whereby Nazism entered the "flesh and blood of the masses through the individual words, the phrases, the propositions it pressed upon them through millions of repetitions, and which was taken in mechanically and unconsciously" (25). The mechanization in, of, through the language is one of Klemperer's themes. "Whilst stressing the organic and natural growth it is at the same time swamped by mechanistic expressions" or, better yet, terms "combining the mechanical and the organic" (30).

Interpreting the creed in the screed, Klemperer excels at narrating scenes of the Nazi mystery that proved inseparable from certain phrases and words like "Ich glaube an ihn" (I believe in him), "durchleben" (to live or go through something) and "Endsieg" (ultimate or final victory).[5] Other words were overused and their meanings stretched to accommodate the new horizon line of affirmation: "fanatisch" (fanatical), "aufziehen" (hoisting or winding), "Erlebnis" (eventful experience) and "Welt" (world), in particular the use of "Welt" as a superlativizing prefix.[6] The superlative worldview counted an endless abundance but at the same time it counted what was on view as unique (245).

> The bulletins of the Third Reich… start off in a superlative mode from the very outset and then, the worse the situation, the more they overdo it, until everything becomes literally measureless. (202)

These news briefs showed little continuity with the sobriety and neutrality of memos from the front during World War One. The disciplined exactitude of military discourse was superlativized into something "fantastic" and "fairy-tale like" (202).

The counterintuitive overuse not of the exclamation point but instead of "ironic" quotation marks beckons toward the Berlin I of the *Sturm* that Klemperer is unable to integrate in his understanding of the Nazi lingo.[7] The abbreviations and acronyms that were already basic to military discourse in the war before permeate the conspiratorial fluidum of the LTI: "the short designation for the technical apparatus and for the group, the secret word as protection on the outside and as solidarity or togetherness on the inside."[8]

In his letter to his colleague Krauss (dated March 15, 1948), Klemperer asks if the copy of his *LTI* has arrived yet, and then: "Curious coincidence the similarity of the titles PLN – LTI, although neither knew anything about the other. But it was in the air."[9] Krauss, however, situated the discourse of abbreviations within a different inheritance. The foreshortening of language comes out of the in-group formations of adolescent psychology, the *Heimat* of all jargon. It was in the heir. In his reading of the language of the Third Reich, published the same year as *LTI*, "Über den Zustand unserer Sprache" (On the Condition of Our Language), Krauss emphasizes the teen gadget-loving aspect and input that fostered mass identification in, through, and for its idiom.

When Klemperer died in 1960, it was up to Krauss to write the obituary. He wrapped his colleague's life around his many academic writings and achievements but didn't even mention *LTI*.[10] Klemperer's indignation over the way the language of the Third Reich degraded "people to the status of machines" (145) overlooks the upgrade in humorous adjustment to the real situation, which, according to Krauss, the emo teens in the army now could recognize or see through. Their perspective is only touched on in Klemperer's affirmation of the untamable wit of the Berliner (116).[11] And yet he does set the placeholder for the missing teens and their slang when he addresses a mistake that has the effect of creative paranomasia. The spread of "sonnig" (sunny) as quintessential trait of the new Germans rebounds from the song "Sonny Boy." The male child who turns gray skies blue lets the Sunny also rise and it's the slip that gets translated into German. This is folk etymology (*Volksetymologie*), a pocket that in the German language collects misapprehended foreign words, strong mistakes that become mint coinage, like "sweet shirt" and "save sex."

Krauss underscores that the Nazis deployed the experience and technique of advertising campaigns and works through this opening into the Nazi linguistic sensibility in an image-rich language all his own.[12] This is the basic structure of his reading of at least two languages of the Third Reich (both in this article and in *PLN*). First there is a propagandistic PR-style strategy taking the form of a discourse of phrases. Accidentally on purpose, however, the larger presentation attracts like a larger marine animal its sucker fish teens or emo-teens imbuing the master discourse with the farce or force of a witty sensibility and slang, and giving it in this way, paradoxically or dialectically, a measure of vitality and authenticity.

Nazi slogans were less commands and more suggestive spots addressing the whole person. Where a command would suffice, the use of slogans would be ridiculous. But you can't command the use of vast amounts of a certain brand of detergent – nor that one work for the common good. Advertising regulates the use of a product independently of the needs of the consumers, suggestively circumventing judgment via ubiquitous slogans, which strike the attention span like bolts of lightning riveting it to a random point (44).

It isn't enough that a person can understand the pitch: the slogan wants him to come along and join in. The turn to advertising got around the lack of a renewal of language, which can only arrive, as happened with the French and Russian Revolutions, by the force of principles (43). Mussolini's unprincipled slogan that all ideas are possible meant that the ideas don't match reality but exercise certain effects, which are worthy of consideration only as means to his political ends, all of which is rather limited as far as linguistic performance goes (43).

The inner contradiction that beset the implementation of revolutionary means to bring about what was in effect a restoration led to the overprotection of the literary, theological and academic lexicon of the High German language – a treasure that must be preserved by and for the worthy. You had to qualify to be initiated into Nazi German (46).

The *Führer* arrived upon his compact vocabulary as on a cloud. But he required a foreign-body *Vorspann* (lead-in or pre-titles sequence). It is in this space of the introductory offer, what we misleadingly call "plain text," that the youth were won over by the "ice-cool Romanticism of the technological adventure" (46) and not at all by the "homeopathically diluted" Germanicism of the main text.

Like the technicians of advertising, the creators of political slogans remain conscious of the finitude of their achievements. Once used up, slogans must be taken out of circulation (45). The sloganeering that was to be directed with the expertise of a Public Relations impresario in matching each new situation didn't constitute a new real language. Only the slang of the footsoldiers came close.

Even though slang cannot replace the language itself, by its expressive tendencies that can be transferred to new situations it frames a linguistic attitude (46–47). Every language has more esprit than the individual speakers, and the soldier slang helps the less gifted with its inborn cunning (49). The creations of any idiom stay on the surface of fashion, threatened by early rapid aging. The currency of the idiom and not recollection guarantees accessibility (49). Every sentence is fixed in order, accent, tone and modulation. It follows that speaking in argot is more the imitation of what was said before than a free combination of pre-existing elements (49–50). All the interjections impart a unique sound shape. The dialogic filler words and those used for emphasis are tied to "unchanging language situations" (*unwandelbare Sprachsituationen*). Through constant invariable usage the image-like turns of phrase become rigidly adamant (50).

At times the images of the idiom surpass the daring of the poets. Our habitual language is unconscious of its images. Krauss reactivates the literalness submerged in an expression like *im Stich lassen* (to let down, leave high and dry), which spells out being abandoned to, being skewered by a fatal blow, to show the creative contribution that an image-happy idiom can impart to the mainstream of the language (50). However, following its successful entry into the language, the turn of phrase soon loses its image power. Only in the current idiom and in the language of poetry can the power be brought back and sustained.

Expressive tendencies knotted together in the slang's turns of phrase can be transferred to new situations like in a creative language. After giving salient examples of the emo teen argot, Krauss must admit: "What is most alienating about these sentences is that they leave an impression that cannot be denied that they in fact evidence something authentic" (46). In contrast to the language in countless speeches and brochures advertising the Thousand Year Reich, this slang was free of illusion (47). This follows his presentation of hardcopy evidence of the idiom taken from textbooks for pupils in the Third Reich that pitched their initiation into the military sensibility. It's a kind of "Emil and the Detectives" narrative in Berlin slang but revved up for war, specifically combat in the air.

> Emil schiebt die Pulle rein und zischt los. Ein Jäger setzt sich hinter ihn, schießt aus allen Knopflöchern und rotzt ihm den Laden voll. Als ein eigener Jäger kommt, saust dem Tommy der Frack. Er nimmt das Schwänzchen hoch und geht türmen, um nicht abgeknipst zu werden. Wir haben inzwischen unsere Eier gelegt und fahren nach Hause. Da meckert der rechte Motor, dann kotzt und schließlich verreckt er. (46)

> Emil steps on the gas (literally, shoves in the booze) and zips off. A hunter sits down behind him, shoots out of all buttonholes and gobs up the store. When a hunter of one's own arrives, the Tommy's tailcoat swishes away. He pulls up his little tail and splits so as not to be switched off. In the meantime, we have laid our eggs and drive home. Now the right engine complains, then barfs and finally it croaks.

In this military-technological slang, guided by a spirit unique among the specters of Nazi Germany, one says everything without illusion. However, given the preponderance of corporeal metaphors, the slang seems more claustrophobic than streamlined: pilots who have been shot down are amputated limbs; weapons are viscerally charged orifices; machines of transportation are organs or organisms charged with gigantic impulses. Men "ride" machines like horses. If they are thrown, they know how to catch the machines and get back up into the saddle. The recourse to animals implies a principle for explanation of everyman's experience of modern existence (in the state of total war). Man is nothing but the staging area of these ever-recurring processes, the carrier of their momentum. The military barracks were the breeding ground of this "linguistic animism" (48), which owed many of its phrases, however, to the slang idiom of Berlin (49).

Krauss calls the language of the footsoldiers essentially a "Landsersprache" (mercenary language), a term evocative of the Thirty Years War.[13] It is not the language of the military's professional functionaries. Officers, for example, aspired to urbane smoothness continuous with the diction of administrative bureaucracies (52). This language of the soldiers is the product of obedience. It humorously gives up as pointless any opinions of one's own regarding the course of world events.

In the fatalistic understanding of the uprooted, survival became a secret science and the mercenary language its compass. But this jargon of the Third Reich went beyond suspicion of the educated classes, refusing to subscribe to the value or verity of all public discourse and its official worldview (53–54). Through a feeling of secret superiority based on fatalistic skepticism the language conferred a kind of invulnerability, which explains why it outlived the Reich to flourish in the postwar period among the deracinated and displaced. When the child or teen in 1946 addresses his parents with the same phrases of superior skepticism, he is not provoking his parents but trying instead to make them his close comrades or Oedi-pals (55). It reflects the stubborn conviction that peace continues the general state of war that life wages against the individual only by other means.

Krauss wagers that it will be easier to denazify language than the people themselves (55). Nazi words can't hide and there aren't any in the *Landsersprache*. The idiom lives on as an argot of authenticity that's more binding than all the dialect borders and their narcissism of small difference. It lives on as an indication of a common calamity, of a calamitous community. For as long as the Germans are still postwar nomads – refugees, black marketeers, displaced persons – there will be no way to guide the vernacular in any other direction.[14]

Although teen idiom is quickly dated (49), like poetry it preserves innovation in language, which is otherwise extinguished the moment it succeeds (50). The metaphorical argot establishes identities through the juxtaposition of known conditions (51). Not simile, metaphor rules, which means that those slinging the slang know what's being transferred, both the technology and the animism. It was at this global juncture that Walter Benjamin in "Experience and Poverty" (1933) elucidated the significance and success of Mickey Mouse. The metaphors are signals of the double, doubling experience of techno-animism. Since both parties to the transfer remain separate in consciousness the metaphorical turn of phrase produces the effect of an inside joke. The secret-handshake discourse binds its native speakers within the community it actualizes. It is a language for initiates only – who are protected against an unwelcome following or understanding (51). The reverse image of Goebbels's "community of the oath," the conspiratorial slang milieu of the footsoldiers spoke to the deracinated who have nothing more to expect from life on the journey into survival or annihilation than the provisions provided – or whatever they can rip off along the way (52).[15]

Notes

1 Harro Schulze-Boysen, a founding member of the *Rote Kapelle* who held a high position in the Air Ministry, was responsible for advance information on Nazi military planning that helped stop the German momentum in Stalingrad.

2 The complete diaries were first published posthumously in 1995.

3 Victor Klemperer, *LTI. Notizbuch eines Philologen* (Stuttgart: Reclam Taschenbuch, 2015), 286–287. Unless indicated otherwise, I will rely in the main on the English translation: Victor Klemperer, *The Language of the Third Reich. LTI – Lingua Tertii Imperii. A Philologist's Notebook*, trans. Martin Brady (London and New York: Continuum, 2006), 237. Subsequent page references are given in the text.

4 "The consummate and most characteristic feature of the Nazi art of language lies not in… segregated book-keeping for the educated and the uneducated… The real achievement… lies in the unscrupulous mixture of heterogeneous stylistic elements" (238).

5 *LTI. Notizbuch eines Philologen,* 120ff.

6 *LTI. Notizbuch eines Philologen,* 70f, 58f, 273–274, 247.

7 *LTI. Notizbuch eines Philologen,* 86ff.

8 *LTI. Notizbuch eines Philologen,* 109.

9 *Nachlaß Werner Krauss*, Briefwechsel, Berlin-Brandenburgische Akademie der Wissenschaften.

10 "Nachruf auf Victor Klemperer," Werner Krauss, *Literaturtheorie. Philosophie und Politik*, ed. Manfred Naumann (Berlin and Weimar: Aufbau Verlag, 1987), 69–70. While alive Klemperer characterized his colleague's disposition as more "poetic" than scholarly, which, no matter how it was intended, amounts in the academic setting to assassination.

11 "An ability to appreciate the dubious side of things and a discerning sense of humor have always been fundamental ingredients of Berlin life (which is why to this day I fail to understand how Nazism could have thrived in Berlin)" (82).

12 Werner Krauss, "Über den Zustand unserer Sprache," *Die Innenseite der Weltgeschichte. Ausgewählte Essays über Sprache und Literatur*, ed. Helga Bergmann (Leipzig: Reclam, 1983), 43. The subsequent page references are given in the text.

13 Krauss writes that the *Landsersprache* in its postwar setting would require for its "reconciliation" the long-awaited ascension of the star of a new Grimmelshausen over the chaotic German earth (55).

14 What Krauss identifies in 1946–1947 as a transitional social condition can, he strongly suggests, become encrypted in, through, or as language.

15 The official discourse, which supplemented its broadsides of folksy mysticism with technophilia, notably when coining names and code names for all the missions of National Socialism, ended up on the same strait place of twilight of the gods. *End-*, used in the compounds of final hoped-for or unimaginable dire accomplishment (*Endsieg* and *Endlösung*) rhymes with *Ent-*, the prefix that undoes. That which is *entartet* (degenerate) "undoes the species." Does the slang of the soldiers catch the reverb of techno-fatalism and infuse it with enough humor and cynicism to help the adaptation to the reality of the *End-/Ent-* go down? As Berel Lang documents, *Endlösung* was the outcome of a rigorous selection process that scoured words for suitability as the genocide's code name. It is a techno term for insiders that identifies a problem's solution to be once and for all. But what's finalized is both the problem and the solution. See Berel Lang, *Act and Idea in the Nazi Genocide* (Syracuse: Syracuse University Press, 2003), 85–93. The referent, the genocide of European Jewry, is at once signaled and obscured, but not hidden, because that would mean it was admitted in the archive of the psyche. Under the aegis of psychopathic idealism both referent and designation are consigned to the nothingness of nihilism without, that is, leaving a trace. Was the Enlightenment Project in Prague a contradiction, a continuity error, or does it project the graduates of the process of final undoing, the Aryans, filing past the prehistorical artifacts of an extinct people without affective contact, identification or recognition? Ignorance of the Holocaust is a gradation of this science fiction and, in keeping with Ernst Simmel's theory of temporary madness in groups inoculating the individuals against the same madness, encapsulated the postwar Germans within their next adjustment and economic recovery. Pynchon's fantasy (in *Gravity's Rainbow*) that the destruction of the war outlined the foundations not so much of recovery as of techno-evolutionary upgrading might be situated here.

Chapter 19

Le code postal

Before he applied in his 1947 article “Über den Zustand unserer Sprache” (On the Condition of Our Language) theoretical reflection to the productive split between the Berlin slang of the soldiers of the Third Reich and the heavy-handed discourse suited-up for talking heads, Krauss threw himself into the breach to compose his prison novel *PLN*, in which the protagonist Schnipfmeier invents the zip code (the “Postleitnummer” or PLN) following prompts by ego-ideal figures belonging to the paranoid milieu of state authority and resistance to that authority. Krauss discovered that Rittmeister, according to his farewell letter to his wife, had been rereading *Don Quixote* the week of his execution and that he was thinking of Krauss (whom he thought already executed, already dead).[1] That Rittmeister reading *Don Quixote* mourned his friend throws into relief that Krauss rewrote *Don Quixote* to reckon with their friendship in terms of ambivalence and recrimination, all of which began to catch up with the mourning process once the friend was no longer wish-dead but dead-dead.

Recruited for a squad of translators working in Nazi Berlin to intervene in and mediate the multiculturalism of conscripted foreign soldiers, non-German-speaking prisoners, and forced labor from the occupied countries, Krauss would have known that the postal code was introduced in Nazi Germany to help the many war-time postal workers who didn't know German or Germany. But he fictionalizes its introduction within a milieu of existentialist avowal and aestheticization of the political act from within the language(s) of the Third Reich.

The direct reference to *Don Quixote* is lodged in an askew episode, which moreover lacks the participation of Schnipfmeier, Krauss's updating of Cervantes' protagonist. But formally it resonates with the use of novella inserts in the older novel's composition, inserts that are at times foreign bodies. This interlude follows a big city detective into the backcountry where he investigates the possibility that wealthy farmers are disobeying the state order to supply fortress fatherland.

Given the large number of towns bearing the same name, not to use the postal code means your letter won't be delivered and the authorities can examine it at length. One hot property among the dead letters is such an attraction that there are some who assume it must be a fiction – or a bum steer. A farmer invites the addressee to the wedding of his son boasting that he will stock the feast with the

DOI: 10.4324/9781003797708-24

plenty he has withheld from the war economy's rationing, just as he kept his son, the bridegroom, out of the war effort by bribing the local doctor with a pig to falsify the report attesting to his ill health.

Upon his arrival in Neudorf, one of many towns by that name, the detective wonders whether it isn't another enchanted place, "like El Toboso, the home of Don Quixotes' Dulcinea" (190). When he at last encounters a figure he can imagine from the scene of writing the infamous letter, it turns out the woman is withdrawn from all contact in her grief over her fallen son. The wedding victuals were served up at the funeral feast. "And so, Neudorf was disenchanted back into the greater Halyconian community of the dying" (198).

The official condemnation of the letter's contents competes with the academic assessment authorized by the office of national character study and primal history (*Urgeschichte*), which affirms the bribe of a pig as a sacrificial act (*Opferhandlung*) presented to an angry god who must be assuaged (180). The expert in the study of the *Volk* recognizes (like another Aby Warburg, but in reverse) that in the Neudorf wedding rites the ancient inheritance of magical thinking shines through a skimpy Christian raiment: "Through a thin Christian camouflage layer the primally ancient thought-inheritance (*das uralte Gedankenerbe*) of magical cultures stuck out everywhere" (181).

In the letter, and in contrast to the language of its explication, the farmer deploys a relay of vernacular phrases that pack the literal into the metaphorical, when expressing violent intentions. To issue someone a warning, *jemandem einen Denkzettel verabreichen*, is the option to do real damage to the other party (176). We'll supply them with it, give it to them, *wir werden's ihnen besorgen*, is another vow of violence (177). In addition to the mighty and full-blown official discourse, which can be diced and spiced by a slang of humorous recalcitrance, it's the references to national character psychology that carry forward *PLN*'s language satire of the Third Reich. This genre of study, which hails from the eclectic milieu of psychoanalysis, ranges from psychologies of national and ethnic characteristics to inner emigration, the intrapsychic pocket of Schnipfmeier's affirmation of his schizoid true self and stuck place, which is also registered as a German national trait.

Can we recognize national character psychology as an outgrowth of the German language's folk wisdom and, perhaps, as a more fitting candidate for the German crowd symbol than the forest that Elias Canetti recommended? It would cut to the chase for an understanding of cultural difference since the crowd symbol is but an instance of national character psychologizing. The working distinction Matthias Göring held up between an Aryan and a Jewish unconscious could only begin to make sense for the analytic psychotherapists at his institute via a character psychology of their culture difference. I will glom onto it not only because it is a thematization of my focus here: the cultivation of a German language of phrases, proverbs and literal original meanings. I am especially drawn to it as a mode of recognition of foe or friend that always ends up being about what's allegedly essentially German.

Being a philosopher of the limits of language didn't help Ludwig Wittgenstein when in 1939 his friend and student, Norman Malcolm, used "national character" in conversation to make a point. Five years later the philosopher lamented to his friend in a letter: what was the point in teaching philosophy "if it does not make you more conscientious than any... journalist in the use of the DANGEROUS phrases such people use for their own ends."[2] But alongside its downside as pernicious journalistic phrase, German national character psychology can be of great service in navigating the cultural difference between Germany and the world.

Once we subtract from national character study the narcissism of small differences, it can be a viable compass for strangers in a strange land. I was twice introduced to the still current German word and notion of *Lebensgefühl*, for which I wasn't prepared (there really is no current counterpart in English). In the first-class car of the Deutsche Bahn one passenger decked out his seating area with the paraphernalia of a soccer match, his team spirit expressed loudly and his pennant waving at every station stop. When fellow travelers complained, he both subdued his acting out and insisted on the justification of his *Lebensgefühl*. It was the source and the state he was aiming for and most importantly his existential right. His fellow Germans smiled and understood, especially since he was toning it down. Shortly afterwards, I saw an autobiographical film in Berlin made by someone suffering from multiple sclerosis, which made a pitch for less bureaucracy and better care in her own management. In the discussion that followed the filmmaker mentioned that all she was hoping for was to win back or achieve a *Lebensgefühl* that was her right. In other cultures, one might expect something like "freedom" or "justice" to be invoked instead. But while *Lebensgefühl* might seem at first an adaptation to historical situations in which Germans didn't have the right to freedom, in the case of the MS patient *Lebensgefühl* was a more complete goal worthy of being attained in her disabled life, more meaningful than a more recognizable political agenda. I mention this as a valid instance of the comparisons across cultural difference that can be categorized as national character psychology. In addition, *Lebensgefühl* is a good example of the staying power of terms hailing from Romanticism in modern German language culture.

Prior to the breakthrough invention of the postal code, Schnipfmeier had been busy introducing innovative series of stamps and devising specialty telegrams for all occasions. Most people experience the arrival of a telegram as a brush with death (23). Why not illustrate the message of mortality in the transmission – or give it a musical accompaniment? Why not install a *Gesamtkunstwerk* in its place?

The challenge to remove the rawness of the shock-effect at its root, while still observing the unavoidable compulsion of the situation, and to spare the afflicted not the message itself but the infinitude of intuited anxieties (25), conforms to what Theodor Adorno in *The Jargon of Authenticity* identified as the "racial quality of inwardness."[3] "Reflection about death is... disparaged in the name of something allegedly deeper, and is replaced by 'endurance,' likewise a gesture of internal silence" (107).

In *PLN* the inner reserve informs the view from on high of the character of the *Volk*. "This *Volk* can be expected to make every sacrifice because its capacity for suffering was limited, because it understood how to take the sight of suffering into the peace of its interiority, and because out of this uncertainty of feeling an attitude of discipline imperiously arose ready for unquestioned obedience" (9).

National character psychology is on the detective's mind in the Quixotic interlude – indeed, he has become an expert, he reflects, just by being a criminologist in Halyconia (185). He accepts and understands the central bureau's interpretation of the contents of the dead letter as rebounding from a more primal time. And he decides while in Neudorf to professionalize his association with the discipline by writing a doctoral thesis under the tutelage of the *Amt für Volkskunde, bäuerische Brauchtümer und halykonische Urgeschichte* (Office of the Study of the *Volk*, Rural Customs, and Halyconian Prehistory) (207).[4]

One of the innovative series of stamps that Schnipfmeier introduced showed in a series of living creatures from around the world "the consecratory celebration (*Weihe*) of a rounded off family life" (57). The series, particularly the stamp adorned with a kangaroo, found resonance in academic circles. A national character psychologist composed an essay on the series to advertise a new comprehension of the soul of the *Volk*. Just as certain Nazi German academics claimed Disney to be a German named Distler and their colleagues reckoned former colonial subjects "honorary Aryans," so the national character psychologist concluded that "the kangaroo through a daring act of the spirit (*durch kühne Geistestat*) has become a symbol of a better and more just world order, introduced and ruled by Greater Halyconia (*Großhalykonien*), and it belongs to us from now on, even though not at home in our forests and meadows, in the same way that Shakespeare through a brilliant act of translation could find his place in the friendly open row of Halyconian classics…" (63).

When an air-raid bursts open the cages at the famous zoo the animals are born free, including the kangaroo, but the locals rally for open season, and the non-native animal population is "incorporated" (96). The state supports the diversion, not only for the entertainment value but also on behalf of that inner inclination to find a cozy corner even in disaster. "If at first the government transmitted slogans of heroic doggedness for the yet surviving ruin dwellers, now it fully permitted the idyllic hankerings of the halyconian individual, who still finds in every abyss a blue blossom" (96). Another level of the language of the Third Reich also asserts itself. The destruction of whole city blocks and neighborhoods offers an empty canvas for urban wit: one joker puts up a sign advertising a sunny airy family home for immediate purchase at a reduced price (94).

Through his renovation of the telegram service, Schnipfmeier discovered

> the single point wherefrom all great suffering of a great people could be healed… Should not the public hand rather than exceed the abstract dread through soulless long-distance transmission exactly here contribute gentle binding where

> it was forced to carry the voice of fate into the house of the unknown fellow member of the *Volk*. The system of the decorative telegrams comes full circle as a repertoire of emotional primal situations (*Repertoire von gemüthaften Ursituationen*), in contemplation of which the dignity of halyconian life can shine forth anew. (23)

The neo-Romantic prefix (or *prix fixe*) of primordiality, Adorno allows in passing, stems from the literary critic who in the recent past was either following or dictating poetic trends. We think we can hear the Neo-Romantic poets drinking their fill of the precious but, Adorno must disappoint us, they didn't write prose in the jargon. "However, many of their intermediaries – like Gundolf – did so" (4). Friedrich Gundolf wrote poetry but was the most prominent German literature scholar of the Weimar period. Goebbels, who can be counted among his students, wanted him as Doctor Father.[5]

Primordial experience, Adorno argues, is a "warmed-over piece of Expressionism" (81). Its flair of "handicraftish religiosity" (69) notwithstanding, "everything experienced in primary terms is culturally preformed" (81). In our "universally mediated world" (81), it can only stem, however tumultuously, from "the day before yesterday" (39).[6] "The order which this babble aims at is itself one that reaches for the speechlessness of sign and command… The jargon fills the breach" (39).

The *Volk* psychology of inheritance is primeval, *and* it belongs to the recent past. I remember a conversation with a German woman who grew to young adulthood during the Third Reich. When the topic was US minorities, she interjected that the Mexican Americans must be highly intelligent, mathematically gifted, just look at their Mayan and Aztec ancestors. When I reported this bit of national psychology to a colleague she archly observed, "that's like saying the Jews make good slaves." It's exactly like that.

"The fact that the words of the jargon sound as if they said something higher than what they mean," Adorno writes, "suggests the term 'aura.'"

> It is hardly an accident that Benjamin introduced the term at the same moment when, according to his own theory, what he understood by "aura" became impossible to experience. As words that are sacred without sacred content, as frozen emanations, the terms of the jargon of authenticity are products of the disintegration of the aura. The latter pairs itself with an attitude of not being bound and thus becomes available in the midst of the demythified world, or, as it might be put in paramilitary modern German, it becomes *einzatzbereit*, mobilized. (6)

Summoning and citing the linguistic pessimism for which the journalistic phrase is exhibit A – as well as the reversals and affirmations Benjamin derived from it – Adorno provides the context for his postwar correction of Benjamin, which takes his mentor's work on a mournful update. The jargon of authenticity that

Adorno analyzes is not, then, the encysted constitutive fallout from the phrase as such.

That Adorno hears Goebbels only and not the adolescent jargon also means that he would judge the hope that teen deliquency signals according to D.W.Winnicott gratuitous or, as the Berliners say, too utopian – and out of place in a setting of grief. And so, he reverses language pessimism's reckoning with the dangerous phrase.

> Nobody can write without phrases, and who is true to the matter who is not also a literate person? The defense of this kind of person seems to be in place after the murder of the Jews. (86)

This is real work of mourning. Adorno expiration-dates the critique of the journalistic phrase, addressing and redressing the thought of Karl Kraus passing to and through Walter Benjamin.

Notes

1 *Werner Krauss. Ein Romanist im Widerstand. Briefe an die Familie und andere Dokumente*, ed. Peter Jehle and Peter-Volker Springborn (Berlin: Weidler Buchverlag, 2004), 84.

2 *Wittgenstein's Letters to Malcolm* (Oxford and New York: Oxford University Press, 1984), 93.

3 Theodor Adorno, *The Jargon of Authenticity*, trans. Knut Tarnowski and Frederic Will (London and New York: Routledge, 2003), 108. Subsequent page references are given in the text.

4 In another subplot and another eddying of the language of the Third Reich, Schnipfmeier's grand and impotent schemes take the plunge in the bathos of the regime's language. Once he is in accord (*Einklang*) with his profession (*Beruf*) he can marry. "As the mere attempt to seek reconciliation between two creaturely extremes marriage remains spiritually sterile and dead, unless animated through collaboration in a common enterprise" (127).

5 Gundolf, a former member of the Stefan George circle who lost his good standing over marriage to yet another woman (SG successfully blocked FG's first spousal attempt), referred Goebbels instead to his colleague, also Jewish, Max Freiherr von Waldberg. I assume the star Germanist was overbooked.

6 Writing to Benjamin Adorno reminded his mentor of what they had worked out in *Origin of the German Mourning Play* and *Kierkegaard: Construction of the Aesthetic*. The "recent past always presents itself as though it had been destroyed by catastrophes," which is "how it presents itself as pre-history." Adorno places the performativity of the language and psychology of primordiality on the schedule of the most repressed sense or tense of time.

Chapter 20

The Session

The cover composition Krauss worked on in prison, his study of Gracián's doctrine of life as tantamount to the author's doctrine of style,[1] portrays the life of a mind "in the rundown stage scenery of a played-out history" (57). When Krauss comments on the ready devaluation of what is deemed good simply by turning to something better, we land in real time; "That is the philosophy of *Gleichschaltung* or, as Critilo puts it, the philosophy of stupidity" (71).

Krauss wasn't denying that he had an aversion to National Socialism, one that showed, but was trying to upend any continuity of motivation and responsibility leading to his criminal infractions. Like Gracián he was apolitical, an enemy of contact with the present. "One wonders to what extent Gracián in a deeper sense needed and was capable of friendship. In any event his intellectual strivings did not stand under the protection of a particular group consciousness" (62).

Gracián like Krauss was in the first place a reader. "His literary formation was eclectic. The temptation to collect himself through poetic creation apparently wasn't a draw for him" (59). What drew his critical writing onward is another identificatory stamp: "For Gracián all artistic representation served only to make visible the *anatomy* of thought (this is one of his characteristic favorite terms)" (72). To motivate the equation that he situates between life and style in Gracián's thought, Krauss writes: "The art of exciting suspense out of a collected but impenetrable capacity (*Vermögen*) is a law of style, which coincides with the basic rule of a militant conduct of life" (64).

The autobiography in the scholarly study adapts to the isolation of imprisonment by subsuming it under Krauss's schizoid self isolation (we saw a similar strategy in Rittmeister's prison diaries). The neutralization of the danger of an intellectual's protest and the parallel displacement of the danger to the mental health profession inform the contrast the scholar plots between Gracián and Cervantes. If the latter held out utopian prospects represented by the idylls, Gracián was suspicious of idyllic states. In the world according to him "there is no point of attachment for the removal of the human psyche" (72).

The characterization of the essence of Gracián's style or life is preliminary and corollary to a strategic displacement. Gracián denies himself "parentheses of happiness" on his journeys. "What gives him the human staying power (*Bestand*) is

DOI: 10.4324/9781003797708-25

the incessant tension of the confrontation (*Auseinandersetzung*) with the tempting power of questionable conditions. What we desire flies away from us like a shadow" (72).

> The impenetrability and inexhaustibility of one's character must defend unceasingly against intrusive attempts at investigating the secret motivating force (*Triebfeder*, literally mainspring) and thereby endanger its sovereign freedom. Suspense (*Spannung*) means here to maintain oneself in uncertainty (*Unbestimmtheit*). (73–74)

The psychologist is the double and traitor: "It stands to reason that no one other than the psychologist possesses in the same measure the suspense-exciting talent of impenetrability (*Undurchdringlichkeit*). In him the essence of the world is condensed into a psychic power" (75).

Earlier in the tract Krauss gave the layout of his critique of the helping profession. Like teaching, it is a handy cover for the wish for power over others. This subterfuge is called imposture.

> Through the art of treating people (*Menschenbehandlung*) all power is won. The psychology of hypnosis, of fascination, is the key. It is not important how one maintains a position (*Stellung*), only that one wins and defends it. That amounts, if you will, to a morality of the impostor (*Hochstapler*), of the rogue (*Schelm*), the Spanish Picaro…, a morality of welfare (*Versorgung*) correlate to the hypertrophic administration of an emptied-out gigantic empire, in which the Habsburgs' sun was setting. (65)

In *PLN*, Schnipfmeier avoids the imposture of treatment by exercising his right to "non-resistance," his unconditional surrender to the laws of coexistence. In this way, he defends his characteristic talent for entering upon the "indestructible order of the inner life" (43). Schnipfmeier, who knows more psychoanalysis than he lets on, explicitly chooses not to "ascribe to nature something like a Death or Destruction Drive" (97). Instead, "a whole other series of reflections opened up for him: the divine power of metamorphosis proved itself even on soulless stuff" (97). On his tours of the ongoing ruination of the capital, Schnipfmeier sees the city becoming polite, at once humbled and humanized – while all inner secrets spill out of the defunctionalized structures.

Dissociating on his walking tour of the bombed-out city, Schnipfmeier hears voices, which he also recognizes as the real voices he overheard in the ministry. But as he seeks to organize "the indubitable reality of his perceptions" with critical reflection, he hears what's humming along the rooftop telephone wires: it's the continuation of the overheard or internalized conversations (83).

Following an incident with dogs, the career destiny of mail carriers, which befalls him on the day he selflessly volunteers to contribute to the footwork of the institution he governs, Schnipfmeier's walking cure, his attempt at auto-analysis, comes to a full stop in an ambulance. It also transports the impasse of his life passing before his eyes: "Schnipfmeier now saw all these abbreviated images roll by in a dream minute. His thoughts mechanically thought again what had been thought before" (96). His affirmations of metamorphosis and non-resistance toured or turned the denial of his broken-down condition, gone to the dogs while splitting and hallucinating. He is en route by gurney to the encounter with the psychiatrist Eurylos, the fictionalized Rittmeister.

For the session at the hospital some reality-checking is in order. In his correspondence, collected in *Ein Romanist im Widerstand* (A Romance Languages and Literatures Scholar in the Resistance), Krauss explains that before the war began, he became acquainted with the anti-fascist circle in Berlin through Rittmeister.[2] In 1941 Rittmeister introduced him to Schulze-Boysen (77). Krauss's one subversive activity, his involvement in the *Zettelklebeaktion* (the pasting of anti-Nazi posters around town), didn't involve his friend. "Rittmeister wasn't even informed, since it was already known that he would reject it" (81). That's why Rittmeister thought he was safe since he wasn't guilty of any subversive activity (84). Rittmeister claimed he was a pacifist rather than adopt the strategy of denying any political stance (the strategy Krauss followed). "I… represented my co-accused as completely apolitical characters, who were guided by a certain Romantic youthfulness" (87). In a note (#45) he adds: "I explained that Rittmeister's interest in social issues was the obvious consequence of his professional disposition as a psychologist." Krauss established that he, however, was a "completely unworldly scholar" which helped make his subsequent "insanity defense" more plausible (89).

As the end of the novel nears Schnipfmeier enters his own prison tract. The object of Schnipfmeier's prison reflections is time, how to compact it or otherwise manipulate it. He concludes that there are two times, time that is the avenger and time that is the rescuer. During his imprisonment the stick is wielded during the weekly inspection of the cells, which is so thorough that, if found necessary, the mattresses are disemboweled (278). The carrot is a daily period between 5 and 8 pm when only a few guards are around and there is respite from the restrictive purview (286). Between the shakedown searchlight on the cell and the daily intermission (when smuggling something out of prison might be arranged) we are in the niche of the in-prison origin of *PLN*. Composed under the cover of permitted literary scholarship Krauss fictionalized his recruitment by the psychiatrist figure for participation in a resistance organization. It is his version of what happened, his pitch and petition for understanding his case as that of a manipulated Quixotic-schizoid type who under the psychiatrist's influence entered association with the illegal activity of a resistance group that promoted nothing recognizably practical but instead pure and purely felt acts. In *PLN*, the treason that he carried out and Rittmeister knew about, the doctoring of the posters advertising an official anti-Soviet exhibition with rhetorical questions about the real situation in Berlin under Nazi rule, is relegated to the adolescent reflex response to the official promotion of the postal code.

Krauss writes in a letter that the Gestapo officials confiscated diaries he started keeping when first imprisoned.[3] When he next started composing his scholarly treatise on Gracián it seems his efforts were left alone.[4] According to Krauss, he wrote *PLN* during his 1943–1944 prison term. “The novelistic form was the result of necessity, I had to secure the work against the interventions of the censor, but the form became ever more autonomous.”[5] After he was moved to death row in Plötzensee he applied to the new person in charge for permission to continue his Gracián study (and thus *PLN* under this cover). The petition was granted but the prison director wondered whatever was the point.

Toward the end of 1944 Krauss’s case was retried. While a certain Dr. Schmidt contradicted Dr. Müller-Hess’s diagnosis (which was compatible with von Hattingberg’s strategy) a third opinion by a military psychiatrist was requested. We know that captive author Krauss wrote out a clean copy of his novel in progress while still in prison, and that the copy stops a few pages before the session scene. The original was collaged together out of stray scraps of paper. I wager that the cleansing operation upon his work belongs to the period of his survivorship of Rittmeister’s mortal sentencing.

In his session with Eurylos in *PLN* Schnipfmeier recognizes in the slight figure’s expressive hands a sculptor, not an executioner. On second thought, the executioner’s blade could be the chisel that’s carving Schnipfmeier anew out of immutable material (102). When the onset of a smile trembles on the wide lips and his raised eyebrows form a triangle, the white apparition looks clown-like. His laughter is “ugly and hysterical” (102). Already late for a meeting at the institute, Eurylos, who still must find the time to write up his evaluation of Schnipfmeier, warns the patient that his case files precede him, so, please no excuses. “It is my job to find everything explicable” (102).

Otherwise, he is charged to help Schnipfmeier, although the question remains whether the client is weighed down by any “hereditary” disadvantage or disposition. After the physical exam and while the patient is dressing, Eurylos asks open and shut questions: “Have you ever…” Schnipfmeier answers that he is a bachelor without offspring. Eurylos: Have you grown roots anywhere? Tied yourself? Do you have a true profession, a calling? (105). Non-resistance is just another form of resistance on the sliding scale of psychopathology. Eurylos concludes that Schnipfmeier’s modesty hides a demand without measure (105), and that his tendency in the face of exacting standards to remain indeterminate and inscrutable is killing off his self-esteem, which otherwise builds itself up out of triggered resistances, but which then withdraws utterly and without resistance into emptiness (104). You say empty, Schnipfmeier counters, I say expectancy, the availability for metamorphosis. In his thoughts Schnipfmeier dismisses the doctor’s tendency to discuss “medical evidence in the tense of a concluded past, as if all life would find its natural end in a diagnosis” (110).

Eurylos challenges Schnipfmeier’s Quixotic delusion of enchantment (106). If I lift the receiver and hear a voice, can you or one of your officials explain to me in a few clear sentences what powers brought about such an apparition? Or is it magic? Schnipfmeier’s non-resistance through adaptation answers: One has accustomed oneself even to this miracle. But, Eurylos continues, through the seamlessness of its functioning the magic-mediatic connection has lost its psychic power. Magic no longer holds the psyche in suspense since nothing else is needed to summon it or call it up (106). Even in your own bailiwick, the telephone service, your modesty has you lingering at the level of stone-age thought (107). But a real caveman would not rest until he found an explanation for the phone phenomenon. For you it is enough that it is explicable, though you would falter should you try to conceive the explanation. In the end you would accept that a demon had possessed the receiver (107).

The testing of Schnipfmeier's occult-and-technical-media connections reaches a conclusion: Your job forces you to do what you can't do on your own: to make contact (108). Schnipfmeier issues a transferential non-sequitur: is there a higher power than the discovery among men that they are equal? (109). Eurylos counters that a terrorist lurks in every savior (109). But that's only in theory, at the subatomic level. It is because Schnipfmeier can't act that an empty place at the banquet table of the mighty could be reserved for him (109). His non-resistance, largely his Quixotic do-gooding, did bring him out of the schizoid position into a ready position, Eurylos notes with approval.

Eurylos asks the leading question attending acceptance of a dangerous mission: Who will mourn you? (112). Schnipfmeier responds: Am I then nothing? At least, says Eurylos, you have now replaced your embrace of the universe (and all the Christian generalities) with your grasp of nothingness. That's an improvement (112). But if I am nothing, Schnipfmeier again, does that mean I am a deceiver? So, Eurylos concludes, you still strive for something: you're full of your self-love!

At this point, when Schnipfmeier is unable to answer, Eurylos is described, with his raised-up eyes veiled by his long eyelashes, as a pre-Raphaelite angel (112). This aestheticist prettiness saves his face a second time, inscribing more deeply the stray bit of homoeroticism (187). If he only knew, Schnipfmeier responds finally, with what failing he had to reproach himself. But all this time, Eurylos advises, his words were offered to explain the reproaches that Schnipfmeier levels against himself. What reproaches? Eurylos: Do you consider yourself persecuted? (113).

That the hallucinated voices, which Schnipfmeier identified as the Furies pursuing him, are in fact self-reproaches is the insight that brings the patient to a happy end of the session. But now that he is free of the Furies, of their persecution, he is also bereft of their protection. Eurylos says that since Schnipfmeier is now no longer alone he can learn to act within a network comprised of the acts of others. But where can he find the others? In the meantime, he can hold onto his therapist: whether friend or foe he can't know yet but what's more important is that he can be sure that the therapist stands by his patient (114).

Following the session with Eurylos, Schnipfmeier rises to the occasion of his "revolutionary" innovation of the postal code. His pitch for the reform triggers a turbulent pro and con exchange that churns up the idioms of the Third Reich, beginning with his own engineering idealism, his imagineerism. Whole departments are threatened with closure owing to the war. Schnipfmeier comes to the aid of the emergency measures: the postal code will encourage the public to help itself. Only participation affords the knowledge that can make you free. The minister of police thinks this isn't the time for the slogans of self-improvement: it is time to admonish the obedient to close ranks unto death (and beyond) (120). But here the late-Romantic quagmire we wade through is punctuated by the salvos from a resistance perspective lodged in an emo teen idiom. Like the postal code spreading out from the capital, the city's teen idiom spreads between the lines.

The minister of police charges Schnipfmeier with inciting graffiti-style interventions in the postal code's ad campaign with his own word play already at play in the promotional jingles.

> Delusional thoughts are cast out among the people for their enjoyment and reconciliation – spawn of an embarrassment over the natural claims of human being, and with a spectacle that has been dragged out into the light of defective psychic outgrowth by a capacity for love that falls short, injuring the innocence of national comrades (*Volksgenossen*). And all this in the name of the state! Where such genius is in the ascendant the germ carriers of decay (*Zersetzung*) are also busily at work. (125)

The minister of police concludes his tirade by making the most of the situation: it's time to hunt down all the dissidents drawn to and entrapped by the postal code's marketing. Schnipfmeier suspects that the minister must have rehearsed it all with the help of Eurylos (127). Or is a blood-and-earth lingo shot through with the ammo of psychoanalytic insight the official linguistic stance and understanding?

Following the showdown with the minister of police, Schnipfmeier accepts the invitation to attend a meeting of the secret "Society for the Unstoppable Joy of Life" and discovers that Eurylos belongs to the group's inner circle. A pilot drops a line that is a piece of the real discourse in which Rittmeister and Krauss were immersed: he welcomes us to "the catacomb society of our unregistered association" (153). Schnipfmeier feels the dark glasses of the doctor's direct gaze resting on him. But the glasses are also the insignia of his projective and paranoid propensity to see these signs of Eurylos everywhere. The only thing to be paranoid about in the totalitarian setting is paranoia itself, which is, at the same time, running the show.

The group decides to save his life and Schnipfmeier wonders that his situation is so serious. It's not. However, behind closed doors, Eurylos speculates that the postal minister would make a great martyr and recommends that he be dispatched accordingly. While these words of power remain ambiguous, another remark re Schnipfmeier, which now is quoted, settles the sense. What kind of sensibility is revealed, Eurylos asked, by a decades-long ability to live in harmonious agreement with the regime of the *Widermensch* (not the overman but the oppositionally contrary human) (156)? But we also know, down this hall of closed doors, that the group is just as suspicious of Eurylos: "As fashionable psychiatrist he guarded the confessional secrets of countless patients, the aspect of the treatment that seemed irreconcilable with the disposition of an honest revolutionary" (161). But then a narrative voice that's a reverb of the unidentified Schnipfmeier/Krauss reminds the group members and us that the psychiatrist's immersion in the world, the big world, is necessary to his role as scout searching for recruits – as "fisher of people." Indeed, he brought each one of them into the society. We're in the loop of keeping silent that Werner Kemper identified in the close quarters of confidentiality under surveillance and suspicion. The unidentified narrator concludes that they should have credited him with strict observance of confidentiality but instead misread his reliability as secretiveness, as illicit privacy (161–162).

When Eurylos and Schnipfmeier meet for the last time it's in prison and the authorities want to observe Schnipfmeier's reaction in the arranged encounter. But once Schnipfmeier recognizes that Eurylos is blind – blinded, the doctor assures him, by the interrogation lights – the experiment is ruined. Eurylos is taken next door, and we can hear that he is undergoing more torture. Is it a punishment that fits the crime of his fishing expeditions? The ambivalence goes into the closing fantasy of rescue. Schnipfmeier's "lyrical-monological situation is breached" (299) when a leader of the resistance, Arthur, arrives like a dragon on the horizon "while the earth burns" (299). And yet Arthur was the insider figure responsible for the betrayal of the resistance group to the fictionalized Gestapo. This culpable figure is inscribed as legible caption to the pageant of Schnipfmeier's rescue fantasy. "Was that the revolution? It seemed unbelievable; and yet the moment must come when metaphysical necessity will enter the obvious language of the event (*die sinnfällige Sprache des Ereignisses*)" (298).

Because "the metaphysical national character had already broken with the volatilizing custom" of telegraphy, Schnipfmeier must follow the track of his own inner emigration to turn the live postal service into a container of the relationship to finitude. "The decorative telegram with musical encouragement from a distance was innermost primal creation (*ureignene Schöpfung*) arising from the minister of state's personal portfolio" (23). Schnipfmeier becomes through his new styling of the telegram the regime's celebrated high priest of death. Comfort, he reflects, comes only in groups, the catastrophe format that is the telegraph's provenance in SOS and the news media. "One is much closer to one another than each individual is to certain death" (28).

> Only dying together is bearable… The mass grave has therefore its profoundly conciliatory character. At the individual grave, in contrast, the unhealable wounds, barely scabbed over by the covering-up process of time, break open anew: on the day of remembrance there transpires each time the return of that unovercome decease. (27)

In seeking to comfort oneself – as in the consideration that the loved one's suffering at least came to an end – one ends up finding in one's own survival the cause of suffering.

When it comes to the victims that the state exterminates *en masse*, however, these must be thrown away into a metaphysical abyss that no illusion of interiority or afterlife bridges. Although the state tried to give the mass executions the character of a secret digestion and excretion process, too many witnesses came under the sway of a terror that could only be brought home to them. "Through the frequency of the disappearance of random people the prize of danger could once again make life worth living, at the same time as it offered preparation for the mass dying in the war and, when this really commenced, for the home front to stay in sync with the suspense of the frontline" (35).

Facing death or something more profound in lieu of remembering the dead forgoes cohesiveness on behalf of "movement," the essence of Halyconian thought or language. That it might be a movement running on empty enters Schnipfmeier's reflection that a mass of people in Halyconia lacks cohesion like any tour group that becomes close in transit and then, when it's time to disband, truly dissolves: rather than take leave, the former fellow travelers look the other way and just go (55). Schnipfmeier, however, is labile and his inner emigration cannot separate from the sense or direction – the movement – of the official language. Lying on a gurney en route to the session with the psychiatrist, he experiences a feeling of faintness or impotence (*Ohnmacht*) that mixes with the "sweet sensation of belonging since his birth to a race born for victory" (101).

The members of the resistance group, like the officers who attempted the assassination of Hitler, seem to be, linguistically, cut from the same cloth as the followers of the leader. The figurehead language of the Third Reich is not an invention but is culled from a variety of academic discourses and disciplines, most immediately the study of German literature. The closer Schnipfmeier comes to the core of the resistance group at the so-called festivities of the secret society of life-affirmers, the more Nazi-speak seems to command his discourse. Because the society members really listen to him, Schnipfmeier comes to feel that his world can "draw from the depths and with infinite freedom become incorporated into the pliable primal substance [*Urstoff*]" (143).

When Schnipfmeier first encounters the fictionalized *Rote Kapelle*, we recognize the group's cohesion as an "agreement arising from the human ground of essence (*Einvernehmen aus dem menschlichen Wesensgrund*)" (131). But then Krauss carefully registers the difference. Following an outburst of power theory lingo – "The idea of mastery (*Herrschaft*) is the skeleton (*Gerippe*), in which the will to life (*Lebenswille*) of modern man incarnates itself" (139) – the speaker, an air force officer, undergoes a transformation. "The tension in his face suddenly relaxed, giving way to an unwrinkled countenance of endless mourning. The melancholy that was the foundation of his thinking suspected the optimism of his thoughts. But the contradiction wasn't paralyzing, rather it was stimulating for the listener" (139).

Notes

1 The tome first appeared in 1947 with Klostermann (Frankfurt a/M) under the title *Graciáns Lebenslehre*. I will be quoting from the selection (pp. 11–38) included in the 1983 collection of selected essays on language and literature: Werner Krauss, "Gracián. Werk und Leben," *Die Innenseite der Weltgeschichte. Ausgewählte Essays über Sprache und Literatur*, ed. Helga Bergmann (Ditzingen: Reclam Verlag, 1983), 57–82. Page references are to this edition and are given in the text.

2 *Werner Krauss. Ein Romanist im Widerstand. Briefe an die Familiie und andere Dokumente*, ed. Peter Jehle and Peter-Volker Springborn (Berlin: Weidler Buchverlag, 2004), 76. The subsequent page references are given in the text. While in the military prison in Lehrter Str., Berlin, one of Krauss's fellow prisoners, who was executed, a lieutenant, "had composed on the front a comprehensive refutation of *Mein Kampf*" (112–114). Was it confiscated? If submitted in the mode of petition, why wasn't the author treated as psychotic? The standards of therapeutic correctness maintained by and for Nazi psychoanalysis could not always be extended when the patient was already on the turf of Nazi psychiatry especially during the closing movement of the regime's "Twilight of the Gods."

3 *Werner Krauss. Ein Romanist im Widerstand. Briefe an die Familiie und andere Dokumente*, 101. In the edition of *PLN* that I read it's stated that Krauss began writing down the novel in 1943 in Plötzensee, whereas elsewhere I read that it was the clean copy that was being made there and then.

4 Peglau (455ff) examines the *Wissenschaftspolitik*, the politics of science and scholarship in the Third Reich, in which censorship didn't in fact play a defining role. There were no coherent guidelines for anticipating or carrying out censorship, even in the strait place of prison. Fallada and other persona non grata could support themselves writing screenplays, and Kästner even worked on the Münchhausen movie under a pseudonym (460). Günter Weisenborn, who also belonged to the Red Orchestra, was given permission by the chief of the security police to work during his prison stay on projects that had propaganda value, including an anti-English drama titled "Marlborough" (460).

5 Peglau, *Unpolitische Wissenschaft?*, 57.

Chapter 21

The End of Navel Gazing

Delinquency and GDR Socialism in Outer Space

The reading of *PLN* as the author's strategic revision of his responsibility for the acts of treason and betrayal doesn't really supply what Kemper's acquittal has withdrawn, the culprit who betrayed Rittmeister. Excavation of the displaced and hidden traces of the dead friend in Krauss's subsequent attempts at writing fiction also won't solve the mystery but give evidence, instead, of a work of mourning (imbued with all the ambiguities of real grief). The sequelae of *PLN* carry forward an unquiet grave haunted by Rittmeister's ghost. In the final literary text, a diary fiction embedded amid the actual entries it doubles, hovering over them like a double exposure, pet grief catches up with the missing affect of mourning as though giving the haunting a rest.

In the 1960s Werner Krauss began again to turn the skeleton key of fiction and fictionalization. Like the cover of his first novel by scholarly enterprise, Krauss wrote the "short novel" *Die Nabellose Welt* (The World Without a Navel) in tandem with scholarly work that he pursued openly. In the science fiction, Krauss presents a future world delivered of the umbilicus of family ties. Eugenics, the bogey man of fascist futurism, is subsumed here by what it advances, the collectivization of the siring and raising of the next generation. It outmodes the old standard, exogamy, which passed along the family system like a demonic curse.[1] The youth are alike and incest no longer matters because even if you do it, you don't know it (46). More like eggs than runts of the litter, they relate to their defining traits the way Mr. and Mrs. Potatohead take in their plastic protuberances. The smooth operators qualify for the transvaluation of the species under a new title, the *Homo Appendix* (39).

The Romance philologist edited and introduced a 1964 collection of French utopian stories, *Reise nach Utopia* (Journey to Utopia).[2] The contemporary reader, he notes in the introductory essay, typically confuses these stories with science fiction (47). The bottom line of utopian fiction is the formulation of future collectivities that presage socialism. Since in the Cold War world socialism is a wrap for the better half, this properly utopian wish fantasy is a line of production that appears gratuitous, even senseless (58). A modern reader of the old utopian narratives who mistakenly identifies these imaginary voyages as science fiction avant la lettre is invariably fixated upon the fabulated technologies, which were, however, secondary or corollary to the prospect of new social orders (56).

DOI: 10.4324/9781003797708-26

Where the social order has been progressively realized all other forms of progress are a given. The figments of technical progress in the utopian fictions were often retrograde representations of what the applied science of the day had already tried out (50–51). While the method of utopian fiction was not, then, a one-way intensification of technological life (55), but the longing for a new socius, science fiction tends to conserve the present social order and economic system and extrapolate from technical progress alone the changes that the future will bring (56). The starting gate and finish line of such a journey is dystopia.

Techno-dystopia is the result of free-market deregulation. The utopian socialist state, by contrast, guides the progress of technological invention (57). In *Die nabellose Welt* Krauss doesn't need to add any new technical props to the "storage closet" of science fiction.[3] His only novelty item is that his world union is socialist. Progress is no longer in question and new properties of technologization are not required.

After the terrorist destruction of automatic technologies in the future world of *Die nabellose Welt*, it is the ensuing work of repair that brings back the labor pains of meaningfulness. There is an alternative to or involution of the work ethic in the free time given youth to calibrate the contents of containment. Aliens who have come across the *Luftbrücke* (air bridge) (27) witness humanity's retrograde saving loop through the fallback position of work. Seen to see through human reality to its end and ending, the alien witnesses inspire caution and ill will (18). When there's nothing left to do but go back home to their star, they observe a new taboo of never again referring to the Terran species (120). The aliens are known as the *Hadrubalianer* or, oddly, the *Hadrubaliten* (16), which echoes the unique stilt or tilt in *Israeliten* (another name in German for the Jews).

One of the cosmic Israelites, Sampurok, laments: "Have I not been washed up onto this deadly shore like flotsam still shamefully endowed with the extinguished signs of a former life?" (33). He knows that the isolation of the dying is a boon protecting them against the unfulfillable demands of the survivors, and he hopes for deliverance from the terrible prospect of wrenching returns to life from and for the dead (33). The air bridge (*Luftbrücke*) the aliens used to come to earth rings in the current event involving West Berlin, the battlefield of the Cold War. It also delivers in the alien's name the only reference to the mass murder of the Jews. West Germany's solo course of restitution, which rebuilt Germany as new and postwar in tandem with the state of Israel, is the heir bridge under which East Germany shrugged off all responsibility for the recent past.

In the introductory essay on imaginary journeys to utopia, Krauss notes that the invention of new languages improving upon old languages, which are criticized as confused and confusing, is most likely the distinctive endeavor making these fictions utopian.[4] The extended example Krauss gives is Mirabeau's conceit that a higher species inhabiting the rings of Saturn skipped spoken language entirely and communicated instead with optical and acoustic signs. As with many animals, the lack of speech meant that they were devoid of deception and error (35). The language of the aliens in *Die nabellose Welt* is a "wealth of syntactic nuances" (31) in contrast to human language, which has reduced itself to "a mere system of adverts and pointers" (32). The alien language doesn't depend on the material world (*Sachwelt*), which by its indexicality human language decidedly does. That's why it can't be understood outside the practical setting of human activity (32). Like the photograph you bring back from your vacation, human language points and announces, "I was there." In contrast, the iconic imagination from Outer Space can discursively reproduce objecthood (32).

Suspense is a condition of reading potentiated by science fiction's experiments with space and time.[5] In *Die nabellose Welt*, the hysterochronometer allows mankind to range widely with one exception: because there is a legend that the end of the world is on a schedule, the fateful year is off limits for all visits to the future. But that also means that – in the route leading nowhere that turns evasive through technologies like time travel – there is a finality that awaits synthesis.[6]

The wide-open space of the cosmos is the "no-man's land" of time (20). *Niemandsland*, Krauss's preferred synonym for the "no place" that is "utopia," can't shake its association with the battleground between the trenches during World War One. But longer ago than that, "no-man's land" already referred to contested territory between official properties. Because the land was in dispute, it was left unoccupied. By the sixteenth century "no-man's land" designated territories that were not yet owned, not yet controlled by the European powers – and which could be rightfully annexed and colonized.

By using the same term to characterize new frontiers in Outer Space Krauss summons the prospect of an unchanged continuity between the race to conquer space and the age of discovery. The imaginary voyages to utopia in French literature circumscribe a "*Niemandsland*, a realm that cannot be found within discovered space" (8). Fixated on "metallic superstition" (11), the European powers plundered the new world, wasting it for the gold and silver. That utopian expedition that looks for paradise offers respite from the dreary reality of exploration, discovery and colonization (11).

Medieval and medievalist fantasies about places of plenty were grounded in the Gospel truth of paradise past (10). In contrast, the imaginary voyages go to the future to look for paradise. If they also go to the sun and the outer planets it is to try out fantasizing under ideally unfettered conditions. Krauss argues that the orientation toward the future, which is a recent innovation that we take for granted today, was until the Enlightenment the object of postponement and denial (24).

While in German letters the utopian journey enriched the A-list,[7] the French output – from 20 to 30 works per year – was resolutely B-genre (16). In France the imaginary-voyage fictions introduced the ideas of the Enlightenment to the totality of the nation (17). By contributing to the fall of the ancien régime, these same ideas, Krauss reminds us, also enabled the establishment of the bourgeois capitalist order. "But only indirectly, for it would entail an untenable simplification of the dialectical course of history were we to overlook the mediating element in the process, the moment of negation, out of which a new condition arises" (43).

Hitched to the exploration of Outer Space, the utopian journey imagines what's left: first contact with alien species. In the Cold War setting, the Soviet space program reserved a prominent place for socialist imaginings of what counts as utopian. But Krauss adopts a hard line regarding the final frontier of contact: "In truth the wish dream of an encounter with more highly developed beings is a regress to the inexperienced childhood of humanity, in which threatened life cannot be borne without the idea of a protective overworld and related religious compensations" (58). On the other side of the Cold War, Arthur C. Clarke's *Childhood's End* gave us the example, since it wasn't cautionary, that could be seen to confirm Krauss's reservations.

When all goals have been reached and attained, the journey to utopia flatlines.[8] Freedom isn't so much realized as relegated to being always only a possible goal of thought.[9] Indeed, within the confines of the future, *Freiheit*, freedom, means nothing left to do, and begs being replaced by *Freizeit* or leisure time.

The insignia of Rittmeister's fictionalization first inscribed around the psychiatrist Eurylos are shared in *Die nabellose Welt* by robots and psychiatric patients. The clownish look under raised, triangulated eyebrows is the mask of every robot (24). The unsettling laugh that is among the traits racked up by the key figuration of Rittmeister in *PLN* is assigned to the schizophrenics in the psychiatric hospital. The psychiatrist in charge of the ward is the tip of an inner monologue that sees in the affinity between disease and treatment the very obstacle to progress in medical science. When he dips into the past, from Christian possession theory all the way back to the Egyptian view that mental aberrancy is the break-in of death into life's enclosure (41–42), his thoughts are in touch with the erudition of Rittmeister's theoretical work. But then the psychiatrist succumbs to dissociation, and we glimpse a schizoid personality that at some point his routine activity will no longer be able to hide. "The moment had arrived in which the psychiatrist's mind sank into a bog of daydreaming and wouldn't be pulled out again until his replacement arrived" (42).

In *Die nabellose Welt*, a husband who has tired of his wife, sends a robot double to satisfy her unto derangement (71–74). But when the wife recovers from this close encounter, she can destroy the robot – completely (75). A target or trigger of sexual excess and extreme violence, the robot models the ultimate cure of mental illness that the psychiatrist alone knows how to administer. He can replace the brain with an electric version, which means that before the patient is cured, he's dead (42). The arc of eroticism and mourning passes through and unites the stray ciphers of Rittmeister's fictionalization.

What began by sifting through the rubble of socialist utopias led to a novel about the genre of a certain future. It follows that automatic technologies delivered us of labor and sent us on permanent vacation (14). The denizens of the future must shape their lives out of free time. In such a social order Dasein is a ghost and the wish to rule comes out of far-ranging daydreams (11). Humanity's true self is flexed only by antisocial teens.

In the future, youth is the only age group eligible for election or appointment to government positions. Every politician must retire at age 25 (86). What remains is a mass culture that must inoculate itself against two extremes under large tents like at *Oktoberfest*. In one tent it's possible to participate in contests staging and staggering violence; in the other tent, sexual excess happens and stays there (90). The German word for curiosity, *Neugier*, literally names a lust for the new, the strong undertow disabling the desire to know (9). The beer-tent mass psychology fulfilling the lust for the new is gratuitous overkill compared to what the psychiatrist and the robots accomplish – or could have accomplished if the connection had gone through. The association is so loose it gets lost when the Rittmeister icon wanders into Aspar's physiognomy. The narrator alone recognizes what Aspar's interlocutor in the real time of the narrative overlooks: his eyebrows rise and lock in the form of a roof, taking on for the moment the appearance of a clown (99).

The inserts of fictional entries that Krauss stowed among his diary pages read, write and reckon with his two-timing fictionalizing with a key that commenced in *PLN*. Under interrogation back then Krauss denied all the charges and consequently didn't implicate anyone else (implication implies complicity). That's the oral history. In the fragment of another trial fiction from the 1960s, "Die schrecklichen Kinder. Am Schwanze der Dämonen. Schlußnovelle" (The Terrible Children. On the Tail of the Demons. Final Novella),[10] Krauss develops figures of his testimony who in turn are witnesses or key figures, only one of whom the editor is willing to decode: Zephyr equals Rittmeister. Krauss writes: "Zephyr is a physician; but his medical knowledge, which is serious, is minted as currency and counterfeit money" (149–150). And again: "I have always had a constant friendship with Zephyr, and he stayed on this level, although his valuation of me was subject to the most ridiculous fluctuations. Usually he found me abject, but on occasion he saw me as somewhat heroic" (150). The narrator, who is closest to Krauss, recalls how Zephyr was summoned to bring him back from the inert condition in which he was discovered one morning, manifesting severe symptoms of poisoning (161). But in this fiction or fantasy, the Krauss figure resents Rittmeister/Zephyr for bringing his satisfying day spent with the dead to an end. "My gratitude to Zephyr was moderate" (162).

Notes

1 Werner Krauss, *Die nabellose Welt*, ed. Elisabeth Fillmann and Karlheinz Barck (Berlin: BasicDruck, 2001). Subsequent page references are given in the text.
2 Werner Krauss, "Überblick über die Französischen Utopien von Cyrano de Bergerac bis zu Étienne Cabet," *Reise Nach Utopia. Französische Utopien aus drei Jahrhunderten*, ed. Werner Krauss (Berlin: Rütten & Loening, 1964), 5–59. Wolfgang Techtmeier translated the stories into German.
3 Elisabeth Fillmann, "Zur Entstehungsgeschichte der Nabellosen Welt," in Werner Krauss, *Die nabellose Welt*, 143–159.
4 Werner Krauss, "Überblick über die Französischen Utopien von Cyrano de Bergerac bis zu Étienne Cabet," 31.
5 From a 1966 letter, Fillmann, 149.
6 In the first volume of my *Critique of Fantasy*, I spend quality time with D.W. Winnicott's two approaches to fantasying or daydreaming as manic defense and to the treatment of ensuing dissociations through the finite/finitude structure of the analysis itself.
7 Krauss refers to the German literary tradition of the *Staatsromane*.

8 Fillmann, 152.
9 Karlheinz Barck, "Abschied vom Utopischen?" in *Die nabellose Welt*, 123–134; here: 128.
10 In Werner Krauss, *Vor gefallenem Vorhang. Aufzeichnungen eines Kronzeugen des Jahrhunderts*, ed. Manfred Naumann (Frankfurt a/M: Fischer Taschenbuch Verlag, 1995), 149–162. Included in this collection is a 1943 poem, "Im Pneuma Münchens," 93–95, that foregrounds Zephyr in the first threesome involving Krauss and Dunja (Ella Wiegand). As in the novella, the Zephyr figure is magical and able to guide the "I" into the unknown. Just the same, the "I" senses the broken, weakened psychic foundation of Zephyr's talents. The coupling that Rittmeister initiated betrays Zephyr. And the couple failing to make him their Ariel left him hanging as a Satan without an inner calling. Rittmeister introduced his shy friend to the two women with whom the scholar succeeded in becoming intimately involved.

Chapter 22

Counterfeit Selves

Werner Krauss entrusted *Der Fälscher. Drei blasphemische Dialoge* (The Counterfeiter. Three Blasphemous Dialogues) to his friend Ruth-Eva Schultz-Seitz, who published it in her press in 1984. On the back cover of the pamphlet Schultz-Seitz writes authoritatively that it concludes Krauss's literary trilogy, which began with *PLN. The Passions of the Halyconian Soul*, continued in the science fiction novella *The World Without a Navel*, which she identifies as yet to be published but treats as finished. She declares that all three works are close to farce, tributes to Krauss's first big literary experience at age five: a German adaptation of Carlo Collodi's *Adventures of Pinocchio*. While the first two works are surreal and rich in symbols, she writes, *The Counterfeiter* appears to be the "first apparently realistic work by Werner Krauss, in which the truth is veiled in a manner all its own."

> For example, the psychiatrist in the play: he repeats always the same diagnoses even when he hasn't even seen the patient… Is it realistic to assume that one and the same person could only repeat himself and never repeat himself?

Schultz-Seitz accords the psychiatrist the status of ghost. Although there's indeed no good reason for his summons at the end of *The Counterfeiter* (a call to the police would have been in order), the psychiatrist makes his entrance less as ghost but more, like in a morality play, as the allegorical figuration either of the Devil or Death.

In the *Vorspruch*, a prologue that is like an unidentified voice-over, there's an overdetermined reference to Jean Genet. In the listing of absentminded gestures that in Krauss's drama are flexed in the scene of writing or thinking, like cleaning out earwax with a pen, Genet provides the reflex of spitting, in fact a particular way of doing it, which the French author first observed in a criminal he loved.[1] In *The Interpretation of Dreams*, Freud says that when German speakers dream of *Spucken* (spitting), they have summoned unconsciously as well its near-miss double: *Spuken*, spooking or haunting.

In the prologue bearing the subtitle "On Dialogues, on Freedom and Compulsion in Conducting Dialogue, and on the Monologue in Drama," the voice-over proffers that if these meager dialogues have offended, then, through this reflection

DOI: 10.4324/9781003797708-27

on language, all is mended. If then, only a few intimations and lightning-fast gestures in passing have given a sense of the being of the dramatic figures, then the attenuating circumstance is the lack of a prosody for scoping out "the relevance and destinal power of the German adverbs" (1). The conjunctive adverbs, Grimmelshausen already lamented, are the wares of Satan. "Mastery of this keyboard of adverbs would become the secret power of Thomas Mann's prose" (1).

The voice-over shifts upward to survey the larger formal setting of *The Counterfeiter*. "For the divine and mathematical language there's naturally only yes and no… But in other realms, it's not the alternative of yes and no that rules but rather yes/no and no/yes, including all possible nuances and modulations" (1). In this "benign climate, our microwords flourish, these insect-like word-formations and word-bacilli, which by their tininess hide the secret omnipotence they wield over our language" (1). It's hard to believe that "all the guiding and ruling potentates of real linguistic sentences" depend on this creepy-crawly swarm of words. "We're bracketing out the beggar's soup of paper sentences, which nourishes only neopositive logicians, structuralists, and other fans of philosophical despair" (1).

When the infested swamp of parts of speech gives way to the play, we recognize in Nikomedes, the protagonist on stage preparing to write his morning pensum, a narcissist of language. He describes the onset of a thought process in physical terms, running the gamut of regression to male birth: "indescribable pains" arise whenever "new life" is knocking. "To be sure, the topic will present itself from a new side! No longer shall it escape me" (6). We never witness him writing. He's always only preparing to write or lamenting that disturbances prevent him from getting started.

It's time for Georges and his wife Eurasia to visit once again. But this time they brought along Egon, a student of the dramatic arts who is subletting a room in their home. He's introduced as a type of genius, and Nikomedes is charmed: "I'll sit next to you" (8). But the boy is shy or suffers "stage fright" and starts stuttering. Nikomedes: "Presumably a shock experience requiring medical counter shock." He lists the medical treatments and medicines that might apply and proceeds to the etiological profile, which is psychoanalytic. "If the stuttering is a response to withdrawal of love, then it is already the love substitute. The flight of the grownup into earliest childhood seeks the connection with Mommy, who's always willing to hear a symphony in her beloved's stammer" (9).[2]

Nikomedes thinks he hears someone approach outside but it's only Fridolin. Is this another boy they don't know anything about, Georges wants to know? Yes, another one, but he's older than that now. Fridolin was the man for everything who helped raise the children. They turned out, however, to be good for nothing better than correctional institutionalization. But then they deliberately switched from outright delinquency to playing the role of teacher's pets to denounce their parents back home for abusing them. So now, says Nikomedes, the Norns of the Child Welfare Services regularly persecute him (15).

When the children enter, the stage directions focus on how handsome Golo is, his sleeves rolled up, his shirt collar wide open (18). Brother and sister are touchy feely suggesting freely that the rest is incest. When they are rude to their father, Egon reprimands their shameful lack of piety (20). Golo says Egon looks just like "der Schwarze Mann," the bogeyman and imaginary tutor their father invoked to tyrannize them.[3] But Golo takes it back. He's given him a closer look and now recognizes a "sullen young man who plainly suffers from developmental disorders" (20).

Departing with his sister, Golo enigmatically pronounces that the gathering must pass "a new endurance test" (21). Suddenly the room on stage holds the four of them prisoner for the night. The characters in lockdown note the similarity to Luis Buñuel's movie *The Exterminating Angel* (24). The other intertext, which is not declared at this crossing, but which we know fascinated Krauss, is Edward Albee's *Who's Afraid of Virginia Woolf?* – a dramatic work that turns the exchange between two academic couples into a bantering ram of destruction and self-destruction. Apparently, the kids regularly take out the fuses and lock the door from the outside.

Once he realizes their predicament, Nikomedes becomes its impresario and starts sorting through what's left after telephone, TV, radio, record player and tape recorder have stopped mediating. All at once they are "thrown back upon themselves" – but, surely, they have enough to say to one another to last the night through. He addresses the problem like an author or director:

> Only that which is most banal sounds like we really meant and said it. Beyond that *we* do not speak but rather it's spoken in us. As if an author wanted to impose his language on us. A language that is constantly being prompted, whispered at us with its twisted and wilted boxes of periods (*Schachtelperioden*), with its stilted participial constructions and with the endless hobbling of its relative clauses, this impertinent contingent of beggars! Naturally no real person speaks like this! How does he speak, then, in reality? Does he ever speak his language? Is it not all mediated and prompted? (24)

Suddenly Eurasia and Egon are a couple with a history. They dismiss Georges for his treatment of his wife, while declaring that the real crook is Nikomedes: "He filled books with his lying stories painted over with one coat of academic standards" (26). There's nothing left for Nikomedes and Georges to do but wish each other good night and camp out in the room that won't let them go.

It's morning and it's the second dialogue. Nikomedes's wife Anuscha, who was in the kitchen during the prank played by their children, enters the scene, which means the stage is no longer spellbound. It's only after Nikomedes and Georges have said their fill, filling each other in about their wives, that it's clear that Eurasia isn't sleeping late, but that she died that night (34). When the police doctor arrives on cue his main duty seems to be to contextualize – to datemark – the psychiatrist, whose appearance in the final dialogue is so fantastically unmotivated or overdetermined.

In his youth, the talkative doctor reminisces, which means during the Third Reich, he filled out death certificates and performed autopsies on the executed. Now they live in an era of democracy and progress (36). On his way out, the police doctor admits more than he's been able to eschew since the end of his youth. "All that's human is still alive and unfalsified in the police force. If the police had back then been as well organized as it is today, then our Mr. Savior (*Heiland*) could have spared himself making appeals to the people to make sacrifices!" (39).

Earlier Nikomedes cautioned that Eurasia must be covered up lest the housekeeper, seeing her dead, be filled with dread that Eurasia's soul was becoming a stay-at-home Poltergeist. The doctor recognized the occult precaution from the period of his youth and laughingly identifies it as "a primitive spiritual understanding" (37). Nikomedes counters that "we see many conceptions of life and death existing side by side. We would not know how to determine which is more primitive, which more complex" (37). The doctor couldn't agree more and pronounces the slogan-like judgment: "For the tourist industry a flourishing folklorism is the black Peter (*der schwarze Peter*)" (38). Can we replace tourist industry with the institute for the study of national character psychologies so central to the fictionalized Third Reich of *PLN*? Black Peter is not only another name for Krampus, a figure from the pageant of Christmas, but also, and in the first place, the card that must be passed along like a demonic curse, or like an unsolved problem. The object of the occult folk discipline must keep moving so as never to coincide with the faux analytic vantage on it.

Georges cancels Egon's sublet and entrusts the young man to Nikomedes, who exults that the young man "means more" to him "than a friend, no less than a friend" (48). Anuscha assures Nikomedes that "never had male friendship led to anything good" (48), whereupon she up and leaves him to join Georges in second matrimony. Nikomedes is only curious whether she will walk off with his diction, his language, as well (48). When Georges brought it up earlier Nikomedes commented that she parroted him only to find protection in his strong words against his weak character (30). Now Eurasia's departure is a prompt for Nikomedes to flaunt his production line of counter-fiction, in which strong words wrap around his soft spot for deception:

> I will continue to produce what my irreconcilable critic calls "the mimicry of scholarship going under in the worn-out pantaloons of a half novelistic plot." Often, I was reproached that it was where I seemed to accord scholarship the greatest room that I counterfeited it most crudely and shamefully! ... What the public believes it intuits in the mysteries of scholarship and wants to find confirmed in my work. Of course, that has nothing in common with real scholarship. And yet the counterfeiting work of art requires a high intelligence and demands heavy sacrifices... What no one knows or can know is that the counterfeiting of scholarship ends up, viewed from another angle, a parody of scholarship. (50)

At the start of the third dialogue Golo is making out with Nikomedes's new wife Veracia. The lovers' duet ends when in response to her repeated wish to hear that she's his first, the first to possess him, Golo comments: "In this house the language of Nikomedes rules like a plague" (52).

Veracia's three brothers, a university professor, a banker and a general, arrive to decry the low point of her marriage. The professor brother is drawn to the desk, which dominates the interior decor, drawn to denounce the author: "this instrument of shameless scandal and crime! It's the desk at which the hateful subject lets his poison pen run riot" (56). When he sees the new manuscript on the desktop, he volunteers burning it to spare his sister a scandalous publication punishable by law. Golo intervenes but the professor makes off with several pages. The siblings, figureheads of GDR society, leave in a huff. They decry the household as a stronghold of common property and free love and at its head is the "author of works of mass circulation" which manifest "his disgusting prostitution of half understood academic perspectives" (58).

What buffers all this for Krauss is the silver lining in the self-parody: Nikomedes is the author of bestsellers who is envied by his critics. This ambiguity is spot lit from both sides now when Veracia's poor relations, her aunts and uncles, pay a visit and are plainly in awe of Dr. Nikomedes: "a famous man, who earns tons of money. His books are offered for sale everywhere, in the kiosks, by salesmen on the street, and even in the subway" (60). But that doesn't stop an admiring uncle from also taking along a couple of pages. He calls them souvenirs and hopes to monetize them (63).

Nikomedes enters ready for "the automatism of the process that my pen describes" (63) and delivers a monologue boasting how well he fakes his scholarship. By referring to the works, real or imagined, that compete with his own, the bibliography is the counterfeit that authenticates it all.

> What a pealing of the bells of unknown helpers resonates within this index of names. Invented book titles with fantastic author names are accredited through the deftly interspersed titles that really exist. What's invented no professional can know – none will dare to admit what's unknown to him. And so, it's quickly incorporated within a treasure of knowledge and makes its way across the generations. (64)

When he discovers patches of missing pages "amputating" (63) his work in progress he feels the guilt that fits "the punishment for being a counterfeiter" (63). But "wasn't it in fact a service that I made the unbelievable believable, while the academics who are taken seriously are mainly satisfied with calling into question once again that which has long been known" (63). He threatens to shoot his wife should the pages not be restored in three minutes' time (66).

Veracia calls the psychiatrist in charge of the local clinic. "What are a few pages of writing and what is a human life? Now only a physician, a psychiatrist, can help me" (66). When the psychiatrist arrives in record time, he won't let her speak. She can't tell him anything he doesn't already know. She should try instead to follow his train of thought:

> You are a German, little woman, I recognize it in the shape of your head! So, then – the Germans are a *Volk* of tradesmen (*Händler*), now the triumphant

> purveyors of weaponry, now the defeated public-relations experts cultivating the ability of commodities to convince. Even the most dubious quality is hoisted by the trader's initiative. Every success of our industry is the product of the sweat of millions of small salesmen. And here the tragedy begins. Your husband is also only a salesman (*Vertreter*)! (66)

Veracia tries to correct the job description, but he persists.

> I know already what you want to say! There are variants, which you hold to be determining, which however in truth cannot shake apart the typicality of the model… Without a fixed salary and security, what he undertakes is not so easily sold… The salesman is the pariah of industrial society. Even the peddler since he owns his merchandise is more likely to make it to prosperity… (71–72)

We hear the recent past that the police doctor brought back when the psychiatrist explains to Veracia that her husband's treatment will be "archetypal" and "through correctly aimed therapeutic measures the illness can be held up… and slowed down" (73). The end is in sight he reassures Veracia. Does that mean a cure? No, but in truth let's spare each other the "ugly word" (73).

Notes

1 Werner Krauss, *Der Fälscher. Drei blasphemische Dialoge*, ed. Ruth-Eva Schulz-Seitz (Tübingen: Triton-Verlag, 1984), 3. The subsequent page references are given in the text.

2 When Egon, who suddenly speaks fluently, next asks Dr. Nikomedes to help, since only he can help him, Nikomedes laments that he can't help himself. "Why is there this overhang made of nebishy noise and fuss" (10). *Nebbicht* is Yiddish but is also a component of the urban dialect current in inner-city neighborhoods in the German language world. It surfaces in A-literature as early as Schiller's *Die Räuber*. It's the reason some feel that the ungainly idiomatic New Year's wish, *einen guten Rutsch*, really echoes the wish *einen guten Rosch*, which gives the name of the Jewish New Year that the jargon borrowed. Around the time of its crossover in Schiller's drama the old urban language began overlapping with and being carried forward by the teen idioms. But lodged at the end of the adult writer's self-involved refusal to give succor to troubled youth it suggests a midlifer's monopoly of adolescent idiomatic wish fantasy. If we are attending here the setting of adolescence in the postwar German language world, then it suggests that *The Counterfeiter* is the prologue (*Vorspruch*) to the diary fiction, which turns it into a petition before the court for acquittal. What's missing in the drama, but which the other fictional works signal, is hope.

3 In the German language the bogeyman has always been "the black man," *der schwarze Mann*, the only translation available in the subtitles when John Carpenter's *Halloween* is shown in Germany in the original version.

Chapter 23

The Ghost Goes Knax in Hessenwinkel

In 1964 Krauss was contemplating alongside his exercise in science fiction a diary fiction that would address and contain the whole complex of hearing voices that was wearing him down.[1] *Wer nicht hören kann*, he who cannot hear, must fictionalize. At least in the diary fiction the voices besetting Krauss could become a character and bear the burden of identification as and with his dead friend. A "sleeper" hanging out in Krauss's diary, the fiction is also autobiographically attended by the vantage of scholarly research. In the entry for February 22, there is a reference to the diary writing of Amiel (Henri-Frédéric), on which the actual Krauss planned to compose a study, which, however, he never carried out. The diarist's despair upon rereading his own earlier entries, which he would like to burn, prompts the judgment that Amiel lived a deception, a "monstrous heresy," living for the reality that the diary entries alone constituted. But there must be a more "legal" manner of keeping a diary in the divide between what really happened and what was really experienced. "The diary contains and conceals the harvest of a life – it is not itself its harvest" (181).

Krauss split this difference with fictionalization, composing his diary fiction not for placement but for no place. Among the collective societies imagined *en voyage* in French utopian letters Krauss singles out one that replaced capital punishment for murder with a life sentence of wearing mourning attire. But if the obligation isn't observed the culprit is executed – for refusing to mourn (56). Now, that's the no place of utopia.

What Krauss kept running up against when entering upon the science fiction genre was his "incapacity to deal with robots in a fitting manner."[2] Stamped with the insignia of the encrypted Rittmeister, the robots in *Die nabellose Welt* are the twins of the hospitalized psychotics. Weaponized in the battle between the sexes they are like zombies on the target range of repression. While the artificial life never leaves the dulling cul-de-sac on the horizon of Krauss's non-fiction, his corollary baggage, the relationship to youth, could be saved from a dead end. He planned at first to go into the science fiction writing about a topsy-turvy world in which life's closing chapter saw the young growing younger unto finitude. Krauss excised the horror of this slow dissolution of civilization and instead made youth's unsolved mystery a problem for the socialist state.[3]

DOI: 10.4324/9781003797708-28

The diary fiction (never to be published as such, but only together with the actual entries it interlaces) bore in its tentative title Krauss's last address, "Waldstraße in Hessenwinkel."[4] What breaches the enclosure of the diarist is the voice of Dr. W.R., but in the opening entry the voice is a felt absence. It's odd, the diarist notes, that the Dr. who dares to hold an opinion on every other aspect of his life chooses not to participate in the "diary situation, letting it pass without commentary" (56). Dr. W.R. has been the diarist's partner in an "ongoing conversation" that is "only in part voluntary" (180–181). The foregrounding of the diary form highlights Dr. W.R.'s recurring absence or ghostliness, and when the voice comes through it shows that even or especially in the Dear Diary setting the transfer of thoughts into words is dedicated to the other, alive or dead.

The editor identifies Dr. W.R. in a footnote as the double of the writer (181 n124). In another entry the Dr. appears as exacting as a malignant superego. The diarist entertains both identifications to explain the interest the Dr. takes in his life. Is he a "phantom" summoned by the diarist to breach his own "loneliness" (183) or was the Dr. in fact his interlocutor at the time of his crisis in Leipzig. The full "title" of the phantom is "Dr. W.R. aus L."

> In the beginning he drove me to self-annihilation, to suicide. He proved to me that I cheated on every examination and that my professorship was an ongoing lie. He demanded that I go before all my students and make an open admission of guilt. At that time, he had complete power over me. (183)

Although the editor cannot offer an actual candidate from Krauss's history to supply the position of the double, along the lines of the literary conceit in *Elective Affinities* of the intertwined OE, a doomed coupling that supplies the cornerstone of the Goethe name,[5] I would insert W. from Werner Krauss after Dr. and follow it with R. for Rittmeister.

After the suicide attempt Dr. W.R. returned as though to undermine the new research project that the diarist was pursuing. Undaunted by the haunting, he concluded the project with great aplomb (183). From then on, the Dr.'s diminished returns happened only at the point of the diarist's exhaustion, slipping inside a dip of depression. That the spirit was dependent upon his mood swings, which stabilized through his successes, is a wish and a denial. The diarist's retirement is his deathwatch, and the moment of his exhaustion has been growing, too. Where your own death awaits you there are the dead who are waiting, too. The spirit is back, claiming to see through his every thought as it crosses over into language (183).

A documentary TV series on incarcerated felons offers an episode that is the epic center of the diary fiction. In it a young felon tells his story.

> Black safety goggles cover his eyes. The portions that are uncovered suggest that we have here a good-looking person who is conscious of the effect he has. The movement in the play of his lips cannot but fascinate the audience. (187)

The convict started out an innocent, socially adjusted shopkeeper married to a young woman his own age. Cornered by new competition in town he applied for loans to keep in the running, but without success. Finally, when the inevitable happened and his shop was liquidated the proceeds would not even cover his debts. "He expresses his desperate condition as follows: I found myself in a world I could no longer address, and which no longer wanted to give me an answer" (187).

Leaving behind his former life (and wife) he wanted to be alone where he was unknown – the better to operate as a scam artist. He lied to deceive the world he couldn't address and that didn't answer. When traces of his crooked ways began to condense for all to see he moved to the big city. He felt safest at the train station. In the diarist's retelling of the convict's interview no indication is given what the young impostor thought he was doing there.

> Suddenly someone addressed him, a gentleman in his middle years, and invited him to go for a ride in his car. He wasn't keen on accepting this enigmatic invitation, but it became clear to him that every chance at a change in his situation could be a chance for rescue. (188)

Upon reaching the outskirts of town the driver started fondling the young man's upper thigh. No reaction and the driver parked the car. But when next the driver tried giving head, the scammer (who wasn't a samer) pulled out a gun and shot him dead.

> You may well ask could you not have gotten rid of this unpleasant contemporary some other way? My answer: the man with his intention was not disgusting to me but simply alien, so much so that he had completely lost his place in the world in which I after all breathed. (188)

It's clear to the diarist that the young man is taking them all for a ride, beginning with the guardians of morality standing by on the small screen, and he duly notes the "irony" of the young man's confession. The psychopath is the correctional incarnation of the impostor of all trades, as pimped by Thomas Mann through the figure of Felix Krull and further monetized in the softporn adaptation starring Horst Buchholz. The entry closes: "All that was missing was that he should next take his leave of the audience by making a bow encouraging applause" (189).

The enlightened segment of the bourgeoisie stands by a theory of criminality, which isn't so much a theory as a therapy for reintegrating the perpetrator. The criminal on TV was not equipped to assert himself in life's contest. The criminality is the product of a weakness that incites empathy while the period of incarceration bestows the good deed of repentance upon the criminal, who is treated and reeducated for the social adaptation that follows his release. But what about the theory, the why? This perpetrator was unwilling to acquiesce in the consequences of failure in a welfare state, a minimum existence that countless individuals live on and with. Instead, he radically abandoned the life that had abandoned him.

> If he wanted to continue to exist, he had to dare to project himself into a completely other realm of life. This freely made decision gives a meaning to life

> beyond all impingements. – It took courage to transgress the limits of societal comfort, decisiveness to obtain a revolver. The first best victim was, to be sure, not a particularly likeable person who presumably showed mankind only his dirty side. But the perpetrator rejected any moralizing justification for a good reason, for the reason of *his* theory of the act and the crime. (190)

Later in the relay of entries the diarist notes that now that he is living without women, sharing his loneliness voluntarily with his dog Knax and involuntarily with Dr. W.R., he has "regained the powers of concentration of his earlier youth" (190). While the Dr. corrects the grammar and diction of the diarist's thoughts and ironically mimics the tendency to "stereotype" in his formulaic expressions (191), he leaves alone the relationship with Knax as well as the diarist's most recent reflections on criminality (191).

These reflections expand across readings in Dostoevsky and Gide. Gide makes his criminal a playboy. But Raskolnikov, too, was easy to look at. Gide's innovation was to throw guilt and repentance into the can and assign crime to a conflict between generations in which youth flexes the feeling for freedom and the oldster gets in the way. "Socialism today has without a doubt overcome the consciousness of generations but not, however, the individual remainders in which such acts take root" (191). Do we hear a synchrony with Rittmeister's fateful inaugural lecture at the Göring Institute? "The perfect (*vollendete*) criminal becomes the epitome of a new humanity (*Menschlichkeit*)" (195).

When Dr. W.R. tunes in again, he's reticent, even shy. "He doesn't touch the past, either out of discretion or because it is forbidden" (198). The following entry, dated April 11, is like a paragraph from a crime novel written in the first person. How to render any suspicion of him absurd? The empty wallet lying next to the victim makes the crime look like a robbery. In his closet a worker left behind a scarf. He'll drop that near the victim, too, to give a false lead. In the next entry on the next day, the diarist admits he isn't young enough for this. But the diarist also knows that he could do it, only the result would be "stripped down," a "terrible nakedness." "Socialism must contain all this and digest it. The reference to remainders (*Restbestände*) is at the same time an appeal to socialism to carry out the total integration of the essence of humanity" (199). The retiree is remaindering in fantasy his propensity for crime, I mean for youth.

Krauss lived alone with Knax in the Waldstraße in Hessenwinkel. Fact. Whether or not the TV episode the diarist relates and discusses at length was part of an actual series on GDR television is less important than its affinity with the central agon of the fictional entries, which buoys up Krauss's psychopolitical argument with socialism. A woman the editor doesn't name was, the editor nevertheless corroborates, an actual friend who did visit Krauss. Fact. But her brother, the diarist's longer-term houseguest, is invented (222).

When the brother arrives unannounced, he comes "hereingeschneit," literally blown in through the door like snow in a storm (199–200). What's been preserved in the cold is the young criminal on TV. "His flashing eyes force me to look at his face" (200). What he sees is "harmoniously shaped"; there's even something "daring" in the way the boy holds his head. Read his lips! He's a dreamboat and knows it. The diarist adds a touch of criticism in his own defense: "Everything you see in him has been rehearsed before a mirror" (200). Would his guest like to look at some of the diarist's illustrated erotic Spanish books? His attempts along these lines lead nowhere. The boy's "wide-open eyes perpetually glued to me drive me to despair" (200).

The boy makes himself useful around the house and is the perfect candy, I mean, handy man. The diarist likes watching him while he works (201). He wonders, however, that the boy seems never to read. GDR youth answers: the old works teach us nothing today and the contemporary works aren't decisive, don't go into the details. His host hands him *Crime and Punishment* and advertises that it depicts the revolutionizing of a society.

> The will to socialism demands all our energy… The indissoluble component parts, which individual stubbornness won't let go, counter the will but can't call the revolution into question, and becomes instead a question for the revolution, which must comprehend humanity in its totality. The problem has not been overcome but is ongoing. (201–202)

The teen, as cute as a crook on TV, tells the diarist that Raskolnikov's theft compromised the purity of his act (202). He elucidates what underlies the young convict's confession on TV: while emptying the murdered john's wallet of all identifying information (to hinder the police investigation) he also took the cash. Only by turning the act into the German compound *Raubmord* did he become a common criminal (189). And what's guilt and repentance got to do with it, the reincarnation asks? (202) The act that's well executed, well constituted is not regrettable (202). All on his own, the diarist reflects, the boy has arrived at the position of Gide's protagonist. But on second thought Gide's character is seedy (203). "The act… has the undeniable character of personal combat between youth, beauty, daring and a vacuous, banal senior citizen" (203). The protagonist doesn't perform the act for its own sake but because he feels justified.[6]

All the hoopla around guilt and repentance in *Crime and Punishment*, which rubbed the boy the wrong way, means, the diarist offers, that society understands the act and sees itself as co-responsible (203). The punishment doesn't aim to turn the perp around but to develop further the momentum released by the act. Only an already revolutionizing society can identify with the criminal to this extent (203). The boy's rejoinder is "inevitable": Why is a society that is revolutionizing before the revolution has taken place more radical in this regard than society after the revolution? His host points out that the apparent regression to middle-class morals reflects the push and pull of the revolution's consolidation. To this day there is no socialist morality, and the bourgeois order is the fallback position when society is faced with the regression to crime. Rather than an impasse, then, it's a stage or step in the process of progress.

In the next entry the diarist reflects that all this time the Dr. W.R. broadcasts were off the air. By thinking of him, he tries to entice communication. But what could the Dr. say? That he was a "beast" (203)? Or belittle his "hopeless dilettantism," his "incapacity for living" (203)? The diarist asks his young guest how long he's staying (204). Now when the boy goes for a walk, he no longer takes him or Knax along. When the boy at last is gone, the Dr. can be heard observing, "now at last Knax and he (or he and Knax) have returned to their glory" (205). But there is no longer any malice underlying the Dr.'s words. When the diarist decides that it's time to bring this supplement to an end and continue as Krauss with the regular upkeep of the diary, Dr. W.K. presses him for a mutually harmonious conclusion (207). The diarist prefers their near miss relationship as it stands, but the Dr. has thrown him for a loop.

> I find in the chatter the admittedly limited happiness of a fulfillment of the endlessly sterile, purely transitory moments and situations of everyday life. That he can recognize only my active, that is, linguistically formed thoughts is clear. I see this capacity further limited to the thoughts addressed – consciously or unconsciously – to him. He claims he can recognize thoughts addressed to third parties and offers proof. (207)

The loop opens with the disappearance of Knax (208) and closes with the cessation of the voice of Dr. W.R. (210).

While trying to situate Dr. W.R.'s "real existence" (191) on a trip to Leipzig, the diarist disclosed that Knax's life span, which commenced in Leipzig, coincides with the relationship to Dr. W.R. (193). He was the shadowy neighbor in L. who became a broadcasting shadow in Hessenwinkel. Krauss was a serial dog owner, naming each new dog Knax. Fact. This is how one gets over the death of one's animal as though learning that, in the huddle of the pack through which the litters pass, life scores against death. But in this fictional series of entries, Knax is unique and when he disappears during the off-leash segment of their regular walks in the outskirts of East Berlin, the lamentation is extensive and most likely unique as well. In fiction we catch up with the mourning that got away from us until it is double-booked like the volumes of Hamlet's brain.

Notes

1 Fillmann, 145, n. 5.
2 Fillmann, 145–146.
3 From a letter dated August 19, 1964, Fillmann, 146.
4 Werner Krauss, "Waldstraße in Hessenwinkel," *Vor gefallenem Vorhang. Aufzeichnungen eines Kronzeugen des Jahrhunderts*, 179–211. Page references are given in the text.
5 See *Aberrations of Mourning*, 96–98.
6 The editor was wrong when he wrote in the afterword that the fictional boy visitor follows the diarist in reading Dostoevsky *and* Gide (222). The boy remains innocent of Gide.

Chapter 24

Man in a Can

Somewhere between metalepsis and litotes the apparent jackpot for application of Wilhelm Reich's character armor theory, the story or case of Don Quixote, must be withdrawn or extended. Like the mirror in Lacan's famous paper, Reich's character armor is not metaphorical. It addresses an actual rigidity of the neurotic body that can be treated hands on and through acts of training. However, something else was happening with the German word Reich used for "armor," *Panzer*, which rolls down the reassembly line to signify "tank" as well.

The extension of character armor to the mechanization of the cavalry, of the horsepower that didn't suffice to get soldiers across no-man's land, already mixes or nixes the metaphor of Don Quixote's delusion of knighthood, which requires a horse and a squire or stand-ins for the same and flimsy play props signifying but hardly supplying the cataphract. The more direct hit and fit with the Quixotic, manifest in Cervantes' bequest to Flaubert, is a habit-forming literalness that signifies and vies with literature.

One year into Hitler's Germany, Helene Deutsch published her brief analysis of Don Quixote as the mascot figure of a posttraumatic relationship between the ego and the ego ideal. And it is a view of the split-level arrangement of a deflected transmission of authority that accords well with Werner Krauss's insights into the two or three languages of Nazi Germany. In "Don Quixote and Don Quixotism," which she wrote, presented, and published in 1934, Deutsch nominated the duo dynamic that Cervantes introduced as top of the line of world literature's juxtaposition of contrary figures reflecting tendencies making up the psychic whole of man.[1] Cervantes' "Doppelfiguren" (double figures) skip the mistake of resemblance: the doubling in your face isn't your mirror, it's your ununderstood. Her choice for the times falls not on Faust and Mephistopheles, the Mann family line of production for which Hannah Arendt knew how to coin a phrase. Instead, Deutsch augurs a political destiny for Hitler's Germany that fits a discursive labyrinth of false selves (448–449).

When she takes the Don's history, Deutsch emphasizes that the onset of his presenting problem began when he, Alonso, a midlifer, fell for the local California girl. She's a *Landbrünhilde* (a country Brünhilde) and he's no Siegfried (444). Twelve years later he's pining and whining and still unable to make contact. Deutsch tags

DOI: 10.4324/9781003797708-29

him a passive-feminine type, most likely impotent for life, in whom the crisis of midlife heightened his sexual wishes while offering only new ways to unfulfill them. At 50 Alfonso exhibits the typical behavior of a prepubescent boy, while in the delusion that follows so much seems borrowed from puberty (444). Disappointed, ashamed, humiliated – Alonso withdrew from the life that was left him and in the subsequent days and nights of anxiety and depression lost his real personality and became the immortal Don Quixote (445).

The Don is remade by repression to wear an improvised armor. Eating and excreting are now difficult operations in his makeshift uniform, which must be attended to with great care. His high-fidelity courtly-love affair with Dulcinea stands guard over his sexuality, which can be completely repressed (445). All the renunciations that were imposed upon him in the past both by the external world and his own inhibited masculinity drop to the side of the delusion's arc from his infantile past to the fulfillment of a bookish fantasy (in the close quarters of adolescence and midlife crisis).

The ascendancy of such an ego ideal out of the ego's decline undermines reality itself (445). Only a socialized ego ideal, one that searches in the real world for identification opportunities and that measures itself according to standards upheld in the outer world, can contribute to and benefit from reality testing (446). The ego ideal that owes its existence to the withdrawal of object-libido stands like Don Quixote outside every adaptation to reality. With the loss of the object world – often identified in the lexicon of psychosis as the end of the world itself – Don Quixote reenters the child's play of chivalry (446).

When the Don returns to reality from his long sojourn in fantasy, reality itself has undergone a makeover (446). What a boy tends to give up on behalf of reality and manhood was now the new reality of Don Quixote. During his derangement, he twice takes a break from the delusion (447). Sancho Panza promises to lead his master to Dulcinea in the flesh, hoping to pull out of the nothingness behind the ideal figure more livable experiences in deception. But the expectation of seeing Dulcinea already triggers feelings that take his sire down memory lane to his first love Adonza. The power of object love disenchants the narcissistic magic. And that means that he recognizes that the woman Panza is pimping isn't the one. The second time it is the approach of death that shatters the delusion of narcissistic immortality (447).

While the Don is the "purified ego idealism of his delusion," Sancho Panza builds a bridge to reality; he is a split-off part of Don Quixote, the part that affirms instinctual life and the benefits of adaptation to reality (447). If Sancho Panza hadn't supplied Don Quixote his own maternal affirmation of life, the knight's asceticism would have finished him off a long time ago. In clinical terminology Sancho Panza is a figure "induced by… delusion." At once the embodiment of Don Quixote's instinct and his reality check, Sancho Panza's role is to identify with the delusion and thus award it that much more reality value. That he believes in Don Quixote's ideal ideation is the kernel of reality that Sancho Panza provides (447). However, he selectively believes only in those portions of the delusion that might benefit him. This self-interest in turn increases the overall reality effect.

If only Don Quixote had been able to "induce" a sufficiently large number of Sancho Panzas he would have been transformed from a fool into a hero and *Führer* (448). To make that possible, however, Don Quixote would have needed to make more room for instinctual satisfaction – especially in connection with aggression.

What seems to render Don Quixote a laughable caricature doesn't rest on him but rather rebounds from the gross sensual world that is not able to grasp higher powers and ideals except in the throwaway form of windmills, illusions and phantasms. That reality should adapt itself to our narcissistic ego ideal is the eternal/internal demand that Don Quixote makes on the human psyche (448). For the second time Deutsch digs into her article's datemark: this Donquixotism of the human psyche is particularly developed, she spells out, in poets, artists, fanatics – including the failed poets and artists who became the masterminds of fascism.[2]

Those better adapted to reality see in Cervantes' novel the overcoming of a devalued past through humorous derision – a past at once historical and developmental. For those of us who can affirm instinctual life and adapt to reality it is a pleasurable triumph to see the ascetic ego ideal devalued through caricature. But the developmental past addressed here must be further differentiated. There is the infantile past in which one feels oneself to be in possession of all perfections. But there is also the past that immediately follows in which the later ego ideal begins to be formed after the image of the highest being, namely the father (449). The world ruled by a father-god turns out, however, to be a hoax: the young child recognizes while struggling with his own sexual inclinations that the father is sexualized, whereupon the identification is abandoned. To this extent, Don Quixote is an anachronistic caricature of the father in the child's prehistory, the father who, while engaging in instinctual life for himself, forces abstinence upon the child. Any devaluation of the father enters the great "stream" of castration wishes directed against everyone else. Don Quixote can be seen to incarnate this projectile: the stretched and scrawny castrated phallus (449).

But it is in Sancho Panza that one can discern the mocked castrated father figure – the father of a yet later era when the paternal demands are no longer of an ideal nature but are aimed instead at bringing about the adaptation to reality (449). To the son who is spending his youth in pursuit of ideals the father appears to be a self-satisfied, stuffed and impotent philistine. And yet the mother, who stands by this father, counters the charge. She supplements his platform by continuing to support the quest for ideals, though largely those with which she identifies, and which stand for the child's own glory. Thus, the maternal influence reinterprets the idealism by keeping an eye trained on the yield of advantages. Sancho Panza, who concerns himself maternally with the master's processes of ingestion and excretion, is also a mocking and loving commemoration of this mother. But for all the readers of the novel, both the Don Quixotic readers and the champions of reality, the relationship between Don Quixote and Sancho Panza amounts to a pleasurable summary and overcoming of the infantile past.

Shakespeare who, Krauss found out, shares with Cervantes the same death day,[3] fabulated in *Hamlet* the emo adolescence that follows out haunting, unmourning and suicidality to a new frontier of literature, which the protagonist performs but enters only as another ghost. Cervantes approaches this frontier from the vantage of midlife crisis and criticism. Krauss refers to Goethe's wish to understand Hamlet as he was before the onset of trauma (140). Cervantes gives us the backstory. There is the deadening sense of a dead end inside him that the midlifer Don Quixote must escape by straddling the manic defense. At the close of the novel the protagonist, delivered of his dissociated state, accepts the end in the dead end. But from the vantage of literature, the cure, the Before and After state of quiescence, is the ultimate delusion. When one midlifer in crisis forms an alliance with an incipient Everyman for himself, yanking him away from his sedentary lodging in love and marriage, disjoining his words of wisdom from their signifieds until they refer to a private reality meeting the chivalric delusion halfway, the missing place of adolescence has been set. Broken down in the collaborative production of literature, Sancho Panza's discourse slings the arrows of his words of wisdom befitting the compass of an in-group idiom or slang.

According to evidence Krauss presents, crime, in Cervantes's oeuvre, is, like sin, a condition of error, a lapsus of understanding and self-consciousness (163). The misconduct of criminals "is the selection of the wrong perspective" (163). The loop through literature follows: Every novel turns on a central case of crime (127). The collaboration of two midlifers in crisis protects and transmits the regressed place, as Deutsch spelled out, of childhood and puberty.

Werner Krauss affirms the so-called delusion as a ruse for plying an alternative to the social situation of the day. Bracketing out the stricken world of delusion, Krauss argues that Don Quixote is beset not by outright hallucinations but that his perceptions go back to concrete sense impressions that he overtakes and overwrites with rote souvenirs from his season of over-reading chivalric adventure stories (144). In the Spanish landscape, Krauss writes, the trace of what will be coming into focus is sketched immediately but indistinctly on the far horizon (144). Rather than wait for the close-up, Don Quixote completes his first impression with the props of medievalist fantasy.

The hallucination-like penchant for filling in and fixating betrays a "lack of self-knowledge," which "is the source of his aberration" (144). If his character armor is rigid, then it is his discourse that proves it. He swears by abstract judgments on what's right and what's to be condemned and he cannot adjust them to the vicissitudes of human nature and social intercourse. By entering a state of exception (*Ausnahmezustand*) heralded by his improvised suit of armor and his antiqued language of incorporation, Don Quixote animates and develops without further inhibition his long-wasted talents (145). Everyone in his circle benefits and undergoes the upgrade to fictionalization. His worldview has the coherence that's denied the average person in the present tense of ongoing tensions and unsolved problems. Whatever crosses his path is elevated from the random and accidental to the status of necessity.

In the Don's view, magic has set a spell on a world that he alone remembers was once dedicated to chivalry. He is less invested in restoring a long-gone era, however, than in disenchanting the status quo. Every encounter with chance and by chance is magically transfixed and pleads the necessity of his decision to joust and oust yet another agent of enchantment.

Spain became a "road nation" in the wake of economic downturns that cast the sedentary populace out into the streets. The wandering that intercepted wider circles of the Spanish nation compensated for the loss of living values (147). The semiotics of wandering in *Don Quixote* heads down the street of accident or chance, lighting up all the invisible arrows and pointers (147). Chance is the novel's master of ceremonies, leading diverse types from all strata of society into the hero's curriculum vitae. Chance is the hidden divinity in an out-of-whack modern world (148). But it isn't only a formal principle guiding the plot; it's the fluidum in which all the adventures are immersed.

Don Quixote sniffs out the alienation of enchantment in his every encounter. In the essay on French utopian literature Krauss argued that the power of nature is that it can become magic. Whereas magic traditionally rested on the concentration of isolated psyches, it has become a result of conscious scientific cooperation across disciplines. Control of nature becomes possible only under the aegis of the knowledge or science of nature.[4] Chance presents Don Quixote with an enchanted world awaiting his heroic deliverance. "The armored figure acts like a ghost," taking a stand like a "witness from another world."[5] Commanding the present by attacking contradiction the knight errant arrives upon each scene like "a cosmic accident that reveals for an instant the precarity of everyday life" (148).

Each scene is the occasion for diverse representatives of society to make contact, clash and ultimately reconcile as the members of the novel's reading circle. The pub is the hub in which all modalities of transport, transfer and exchange meet and cross over (128). Metaphysical arguments lead to brawling, which cannot but attract the omnipresent police force. It is by the force of a *politesse* transcending enforcement that all contact becomes permeable and productive of more narration. The transformation of the everyday world as Don Quixote perceives it evokes at once transubstantiation, pagan metamorphosis, and the outbreak of mental illness (128).

When all Don Quixote's old and newly made friends join him in avowing that the bucket is in fact the helmet of Mambrino, we stand before a complete collapse of the empirically grounded world and word (156). His armor isn't backed by anything real, not even by money, the representative of lost reality, but only by the unbridled demand for distinction, for fame (158). When the protagonist discovers how popular his history has become because both the first book and the forgery of the sequel are out and they're all anyone talks about, it becomes clear that he's interested in something else, something more (180). The hero disapproves of the novella inserts in the first book because they interrupt the writing down of his action which is what supplies "the epic totality for the infinitude of his subjective essence and striving" (142).

In Krauss's reading Don Quixote's discourse approximates that of the quintessential modern academic. "Cervantes's entire literary formation was… creative literary criticism" (181). In writing about French utopian *voyages imaginaires*

Krauss underscores that whereas today in the GDR literary scholarship follows and facilitates the appreciation of existing works, in earlier centuries the standards of criticism intervened in and dictated the process of poetic self-understanding.[6] By earlier he also meant, in the greater context of his reflections on literature and language, the autonomy in German letters of a literary criticism preliminary to its instrumentalization in the languages of the Third Reich.

Don Quixote realizes the second calling of his discourse – to become literature – through the contribution of Sancho Panza (159). Don Quixote's sententious and antiqued discourse is always preliminary to the deed it introduces and announces (175). Sancho Panza's vernacular words of wisdom run commentary on the deed that just happened. The discourses mingle on the road when their contexts and other containers no longer hold. "Don Quixote's greatest triumph was to hook a sedentary farmer on the tagline of his delusion, to set this bound spirit in motion and bring his valuable treasure of proverbial wisdom into the circulation of speech" (175). The inexhaustibility of Panza's memory, the cornucopia replete with proverbs and sayings, grants him the breadth and wealth of a spontaneity that never runs dry (161). There are no class boundaries in the way of becoming a poet (162). But it takes just these two to fashion the literary discourse of the premier modern novel, which is set to go once Sancho Panza's perspective proves as split off as Don Quixote's master discourse of chivalry. The second hero's commentary is internally askew. On the road of chance or accident, he cannot supply the habitual fit between proverbial sayings and their matching situations and experiences. By following a deranged master on his wandering adventures, Sancho Panza had to let go the link between his sayings and their specific life situations (162). On the road he whimsically strings together the signifiers in chaotic disconnection from their signifieds.

The main arc of the novel is "the power of literature" (167). For Sancho Panza his master's dissociated chivalric fantasying has at least the same claim to reality as his own prior sedentary existence: he rises to the occasion and as the second hero of the novel makes demands on the author (161). The whole novel can be seen as an enormous conversation about literature, with Cervantes' novel in the foreground: "In *Don Quixote* all is literature and all literature is human existence" (166). The knight errant's "deeds are a compendium of this literature, a capital topic for conversation on all the streets he enlivens" (167). And by word of mouth even the illiterate can take part in these literary fictions from the past.

Popular editions in the shorter form of novelette (*Romanze*) had in the meantime mediated the old epics of knighthood (168). The adaptation simplified the temporal mode of all the past deeds and foregrounded the time of this condensation as the space of heroic prehistory (168). Quilting points of this B-literary conceit of a more readily transportable, transposable past, advertised by the phenomenon of Don Quixote, both the figure and subsequently the novel itself, get stitched into the understanding of the present (168).

The fictive realm of the popularized chivalric adventure is a sham past that "never possessed life and cannot readily attain the guarantee (*Gewähr*) of real death." *Gewähr* shares one soundshape with the German word for firearm, *Gewehr*. Over a century before Don Quixote entered the delusion of chivalry the introduction of firepower had rendered basic armor gratuitous in combat. It was a firearm that maimed Cervantes's left hand, which was henceforth useless, dangling like an extra name distinguishing the warrior who left the battlefield to engage with literature. Unauthorized to supply the *Gewähr* of death Don Quixote's performance drops the author's *Gewehr* in the recent past, which is prehistory, and leaves it there, deep inside or behind a new life in literature.

Werner Krauss develops the self-reflexive conceit that *Don Quixote* is a modern novel by dint of its kinship with literary criticism, which is the special strain in his own work between scholarship and literature. But it's also a self-critical reflection since he attributes this stain on the German language (as do Victor Klemperer and Theodor Adorno) to the linguistic adaptation to the Third Reich. There's always one member of the committee judging the suitability of candidates for admission to an art program who will jokingly wonder what if another Hitler has been excluded – another career launch for the politics of resentment. But it's also possible to be suspicious that anyone who studies or teaches literature might betray the calling (or upgrade it) by going into politics like Goebbels.

Notes

1 Helene Deutsch, "Don Quijote und Donquijotismus," *Imago*, 20, 4 (1934), 444–449. Page references are given in the text. Her article appeared in English ("Don Quixote and Don Quixotism") in *Psychoanalytic Quarterly*, 6 (April 1937), 215–222.
2 Of course, there are those who overlook the warning labels and identify with "The Man of La Mancha" just the same, with the avatar of heroism in his striving for the fulfillment of his ideal. The musical dreams the impossible dream, the midlife criticism of reality in which adolescence rallies for a last hurrah, and by equating Don Quixote and Cervantes, situating them in a tableau of faux theatrical improvisation, places reading, writing and authorship backstage and off screen.
3 Werner Krauss, *Miguel de Cervantes. Leben und Werk* (Neuwied and Berlin-West: Hermann Luchterhand Verlag, 1966), 145. This was his second book on Cervantes' oeuvre. The subsequent page references are given in the text.
4 Werner Krauss, "Überblick über die Französischen Utopien von Cyrano de Bergerac bis zu Étienne Cabet," *Reise Nach Utopia*, 48–49.
5 *Miguel de Cervantes. Leben und Werk*, 148. The subsequent page references will continue to be given in the text.
6 *Reise nach Utopia*, 96.

Chapter 25

Don Quixote and Nazi Literature in Kathy Acker and Robert Bolaño

Jean François Lyotard's conceit that the postmodern precedes the modern comes true with the "first modern novel."[1] As Krauss elucidated in his Cervantes scholarship, unlike poetry, which is something like a birthright or at least an accessory to the initiation rites and writing of puberty, prose requires the prep work of reading and readings (or criticism). The intake of the novel loops through *Don Quixote* until all the characters are joined in its reading circle. Although the knight is left out on a limb, the dead-end track of recovery, it counts as a happy ending. Flaubert in *Madame Bovary* takes this condition of literary self-reading to the next, lethal level.

Between *PLN* and the article "On the Condition of Our Language," Krauss delved into an enabling contrast between idioms, which in Cervantes' novel is the meeting and mixing of two alien linguistic sensibilities, the knight's borrowed lofty discourse and the squire's phrases and words of wisdom. The unlikely alliance crosses over into literature by dint of both sensibilities being skewed, uprooted or deranged, like the shattering of the sedentary signified upon the nomadic trek of the signifier. In his fictionalization and theorization of the languages of the Third Reich, Krauss presents the cohabitation of a German-only academic discourse with an emo-adolescent sensibility or style, which is more cynical but just as empty or, in other words, nihilistic. In *PLN* Schnipfmeier is the impresario of the impossible dream of innovation in the face-off or interface between the emo-opposed mindsets.

It is more fate than accident that Kathy Acker chose *Don Quixote* as the site for an artistic appropriation not only of Cervantes' plot points and signifiers but also of pull quotes from the theories championed at that time in the academic departments of the study of literature, updating the sparring of styles by including poststructuralist theories.[2] The spokesperson of the post-punk challenge of theorization of and in literature is the eponymous heroine. In getting an abortion she was christened Knight/Night and her squire, a talking dog, hails from another corner of Cervantes's oeuvre. The *Los Angeles Times* review of Acker's new novel (on November 9, 1986) hovers over it like a cartoon's speech bubble. "She is like a graduate student in comparative literature gone looney-tunes under the pressure of orals." The criticism that is journalism is the denial of a new continuity between the

DOI: 10.4324/9781003797708-30

theoretical study of literature and the production line of novels. Acker's discourse overlaps with journalism (the success story of academic criticism) via the politics it carries forward from theory on campus. If literature departments represented in 1986 the center foldout of intellectual life in the US, then in the review of Acker's novel extramural journalism ineptly sought to intercept its influence.

On the last page the female Night salutes "these teachings," which she obeys, and which are her "last memories" (207) and returns to her signature horse and her adventurous dubbing of phrases. The horse she rides away on at the end fulfilled a wish tethered to the opening bout of paronomasia during which she christened the medical props close to hand at the abortion clinic:

> her wheeling bed's name was "Hack-kneed" or "Hackneyed," meaning "once a hack" or "always a hack" or "a writer" or "an attempt to have an identity that always fails." Just as "Hackneyed" is the glorification or change from non-existence into existence of "Hack-kneed," so, she decided, "catheter" is the glorification of "Kathy." (10)

Henceforth riding means writing and every appropriation is to the glory of one author, the one steeling the feminist resolve to have and to hold an oeuvre of her own by stealing the story of "Don Quixote."

What are the teachings with which she rides/writes away? In the closing section we learn that Spain prior to the civil war – like the US campus in 1986 – was enjoying a cultural renaissance. There were two intellectual currents dominant at that time, in that place. Other than a nationalistic Catholicism, there was the critical discourse derived from Karl Kraus (203). The novel doesn't spell any of this out and after the name drops the fantasy history turns to "Kraus' main Spanish disciple" who advanced a doctrine of "harmonious rationalism" (203). Wasn't Karl Kraus a Quixotic warrior jousting against the journalistic phrase? When the question is raised how the stimulus of language affected Spanish politics, it is never answered from the vantage of Kraus (or Walter Benjamin on Kraus) (204). Like a continuity error in film, the empty citation and summoning of Karl Kraus performs a loss that cannot be metabolized. At the same time, when faced with the Nazi symptom of the weaponized phrase this Don doesn't surrender, as Kraus so eloquently did.

The Third Reich in and as literary language became the hallmark of another representative of the post-postmodern reception of *Don Quixote*. By critical consensus *The Savage Detectives* by Roberto Bolaño stages a Quixotic adventure in which two poets travel in search of their Dulcinea, the mother of their school of poetry. The sequel, *2666*,[3] begins with another Quixotic quest involving four academics trying to find the enigmatic and elusive German author Arcimboldi. The spreading middle section collects the evidence in the race to trace a serial killer of women in the Mexican town where the German author was last seen. The final part, the life story of the author, is a wrap with the quintessential postwar memoir of the innocent bystander crafted by any one of the key West German authors, like

Heinrich Böll or Günther Grass. At the end Arcimboldi departs for Mexico to help clear his nephew of the serial murder charge.

In the tale of Arcimboldi, there is a direct reference to Cervantes' novel. It is deposited inside the introjected diary of a certain Ansky, which the German author as a young man, Reiter was his name at that time, discovered while soldiering in a stretch of Eastern Europe. The diarist had already been liquidated together with the rest of the Jewish population. Reiter memorizes or incorporates the pages, which continue to turn following his sudden resolve to write literature. The name doesn't ride or write him because he's not at home in the Oedipus complex but like the two protagonists of P.K. Dick's *Martian Time-Slip* is suspended between autism and schizophrenia. His vacancy acts as inoculation against the psychopathic idealism of National Socialism. But lacking any resonance in the emptiness for the direct hit of his name, he takes a nom de plume from Ansky's diary, who celebrates Arcimboldi's paintings "as happiness personified. The end of semblance" (734).

Inside this foreign deposit, which we join Reiter in reading or recalling, Ansky at one point befriends a Soviet writer, Ivanov, and imparts to him the authorship enzyme that the diary bestows on Reiter. He dictates a science fiction that brings the writer a season of fame. The novel is touted as "the Don Quixote of Soviet science fiction" (723). "Ivanov considered himself the Cervantes of fantastic literature" rather than another knight errant because he "saw only himself riding alongside a mysterious and indispensable Sancho across the steppes of literary glory" (723). After the third novel, however, all his work is withdrawn from the bookstores, and he is expelled from the party. During the show trial, which ends in his execution, Ivanov, as Ansky underscores, never betrayed their Panza scheme: "Accomplices in imposture until the end" (731). Stepping to the side of his incorporation of the diary, Reiter sees "a column of German tanks moving east. They looked like the coffins of an extraterrestrial civilization" (740).

Ansky's reflections on semblance also continue in Reiter's words, which the soldier applies to his being in the Third Reich, novelizing it as Krauss did in *PLN*.

> Semblance was an occupying force of reality… even the most extreme, borderline reality. It lived in people's souls and their actions, in willpower and in pain, in the way remorse and priorities were ordered… National Socialism was the ultimate realm of semblance… Youth is the semblance of strength; love is the semblance of peace. (741)

Can "is the semblance of" be other words for "is the synonym for"?

Arcimboldi writes his first novel in postwar Cologne, but to prepare his manuscript for submission he needs a typewriter, which he rents from an older gent whose discourse on the interrelation between minor works and masterpieces is the only other deposit in the vacuity of the author's schizoid or autistic state. It also maps onto the dialectic of the two authors and two languages of *Don Quixote*.

"Every minor work has a secret author, and every secret author is, by definition, a writer of masterpieces" (785). What you see watching over his shoulder while the writer writes is a "semblance," a "shell of literature… The person who really writes the minor work is a secret writer who accepts only the dictates of a masterpiece" (786).

> There's nothing inside the man who sits there writing. Nothing of himself, I mean… He writes like someone taking dictation… Every work that isn't a masterpiece is, in a sense, a part of a vast camouflage… Every work that isn't a masterpiece is cannon fodder, a slogging foot soldier, a piece to be sacrificed, since in multiple ways it mimics the design of the masterpiece. (786)

All minor works can be nothing but plagiarism of some masterpiece. But this is sanctioned plagiarism, camouflage like some wood and canvas scenery. It is a "charade that leads us, likely as not, into the void" (787). The owner of the typewriter manages to fit the languages of the Third Reich as explored by Krauss inside the scene of writing minor and/or great literature.

Why doesn't Arcimboldi start with poetry? He is convinced that "all poetry, of any style, was contained or could be contained in fiction" (774). A German author running on the incorporation of alien words inside a basic void, depositing the found wordage as placeholders for the novels to come, is the cartoon reversal of Bolaño's own slow-mo metabolization of prose out of poetry, academic criticism and review journalism. He was for decades doing the limbo with the half-educated poets who occupy the foreground of his narrative retrospective. While in my research archive everyone is immersed in psychoanalysis, in the fictive world of Bolaño's novels everyone is a poet. He saved up his prose-writing-self for a stretch (around a decade) of composing highly readable novels, two of them gigantic.

Bolaño heard National Socialism resound in the violent overthrow of Allende and Pinochet's takeover. But the pages in Germany's open book of evil politics turned toward other facets of Germanicity under Bolaño's aegis. The general human condition of poetry forged a notion of Nazi literature. The first-person narrator of *By Night in Chile*,[4] a priest whose breakthrough experience, however, was getting to know the country's leading literary critic, is himself a critic and a poet, who climbs to the top of the superstructure under Pinochet. At a gathering of writers which the literary critic regularly hosts, an older poet recounts his meeting with Ernst Jünger in Nazi-occupied Paris. Their exchange passed through an elevated academic discourse checking off the themes home on the range of conversation with a figurehead of the Third Reich.

> Far from the idle but agitated and often indiscreet chatter of the Parisian salons, the Chilean writer and the German writer enjoyed a free-ranging conversation, touching on the human and the divine, war and peace, Italian painting and Nordic painting, the source of evil and the effects of evil that sometimes seem to be triggered by chance, the flora and fauna of Chile, which Jünger seemed to have read about in the works of his fellow countryman Philippi, who was at once a true Chilean and a true German. (32)

If there is a high point in the priest-narrator's upward mobility following the fall of Allende it is his commission to teach the generals running Chile's dictatorship all about Marxism. The seminar seems an exercise in the manner of psychological warfare developed between the world wars in Germany on a Freudian basis. The seminar participants are studying the enemy from the distance of their resolute and intact vantage, which they flex as superiority in word power.

> In the third class we returned to the Manifesto. According to General Leigh it was an unadulterated urtext. He didn't elaborate. At first, I thought he was making fun of me, but it soon became clear that he was serious. I'll have to think about that later, I said to myself. (84)

Like the staggered way in which the influence of found wordage imparts itself to Arcimboldi, each of the seminar exchanges is set up in three phases: there is a fascist and his language, then the priest comes under the influence, and finally that influence inscribes itself in the narrative. The priest has included among the assigned readings one text on Marx by a female Chilean academic who studied abroad with Althusser. The generals are more interested in her own political and sexual leanings, which they characterize in a misogynistic manner not expected in polite society. When it becomes clear that the "bitch" is being watched and will be taken care of the sooner the better, the priest makes mental notes for a poem he is inspired to write about a fallen woman (86–87). Pinochet rails against the myth that Allende was a cultured intellectual, claiming that while he has published three books on military history and strategy, the fraud hardly read and didn't publish. The priest follows his lead and owns it: "I always suspected as much I whispered" (90). In the session dedicated to Friedrich Engels' treatise on the family and private property, the alternation between the priest's instruction and the dictator nodding and asking "pertinent questions" culminates in the view enjoyed by the duo. What does the schizoid see when he looks up at the heavens as though inspired rather than lock gazes during a toast? It is a horizon line pulled out of science fiction. "And from time to time both of us fell silent and looked at the moon sailing on alone through infinite space" (85).

Science fiction affords a faux poetic license where aestheticization of politics is de rigeur. In *Nazi Literature in the Americas* and *Distant Star* the Chilean sky-writing artist of death, Ramirez Hoffman, is not a poet but a criminal, says the author's representative in the fictive account he narrates.[5] There are serial killers who see themselves as artists without any national, ideological, or group motivation. Charged as a torturer after the regime change, Hoffman publishes unrepentant rationalizations joining Amilcar Lobo on the dark side of politics. This is where the detective Romero and the unnamed narrator conspire to track him down decades after his exhibition of the snuff photos of his victims. The narrator finds two publications that by their "singularity of purpose" set them apart from the rest of the rightwing press, which packs away case study "material for a variegated sampler of psychopathy and schizophrenia" (130). Walking the flat line between the fateful profundity of nihilism and its cynical celebration, the Chilean poet, by another name, "argued that literature should be written by non-literary people, just as politics should be and indeed was being taken over by non-politicians" (135). Literature will be abolished when poetry written by non-poets is read by non-readers (135). Implicated in the detective's execution of Hoffman in Bolaño's adopted town, the narrator is appalled by "literature's bottomless cesspools" (130) and resolves to go back to being an unpublished poet working a day job.

The more legible doubling lies between the narrator and the detective. Bolaño delighted in pronouncing in interviews his wish to be a criminal investigator cutting to the chase, cutting through the layering of undecidability, to the guilt and past it. It is when their exchange illuminates their incompatibility that we learn more about the author. The detective conjures the interest that an exceptional character holds for him: "He's like a session with a psychoanalyst, Romero said. It was immediately clear to me that he had never undergone psychoanalysis, although it was a form of treatment for which he had the highest regard" (119). Other references to psychoanalysis in Bolaño's fiction, which are few and far between, are equally circumspect and implicit. And yet we sense that its highest regard entered the staging of his turn to prose in *The Third Reich.*

Moving to Europe and finally settling on the Spanish coast, Bolaño witnessed the German tourism industry sending history on vacation, making travel plans that reversed the old retreat and defeat. *The Third Reich*, which he wrote in 1989, may have been his first exercise in writing the readable prose that carried him forward for around a decade.[6] Did he intend to publish it down the road or was it to remain an exercise, a sacrifice secretly lodged in the foundation of all that followed? That the end remains unfinished can also mean that all that followed was the search for this ending.

There was another end that was not addressed in the 1989 novel, namely, the fall of the wall. Does the conceit of the war strategy game almost require the Cold War vantage on the recent past? Ian Fleming wrote the epic adventures of James Bond on the crypt of World War Two, which the Cold War opposition blocked from view or denied. Out of the crypt he drew the underworld organization suitably named SPECTRE as third-party parasite of the dyadic stalemate. Hostilities were contained in a board game played by the ghosts of both perpetrators and victims from the recent past of the Third Reich.[7]

There is the legend that Mrs. Heidegger, upon delivering her husband by car to the conference center in Normandy, exclaimed to the welcoming hosts: What a great *Autobahn* we built for you! Did Fortress Europe lay the infrastructure for the postwar European Union, in which, peekaboo, German power continued to hide out? That the novel's title is the name of the grand war strategy game, which the protagonist, the oblivious German tourist Udo Berger, takes along with him on his vacation, performs the condition of not-seeing triggering his hallucinatory peripheral vision.

In German, a game is "play" (*Spiel*), a term central to the typology of drama, from *Lustspiel* or comedy to *Trauerspiel* or tragedy. Looking at the game from both sides now, both the psychotic and the creative sides in the close quarters of traumatic history, describes the *Spiel* that Bolaño's prose would follow out. Given the central mystery of contemporary German literature in the literary cosmos he projected in Spain, this first document might suggest that he started out identifying with German culture's knack for game changing. More specifically in the case of Bolaño, it is the knack for identifying with a lost cause that modeled a strategy for surviving poetry in prose.

That the game holds the place of poetry is hinted at on a few occasions. If the equation cannot in fact be drawn since there can be no poetry after Auschwitz, then the game's match with traumatic history can be seen as the postmodern circumnavigation of the prohibition. Upon arriving in Spain Berger decides to start keeping a diary, which completes the scene of writing by putting him on the track of the author's own decision to write prose rather than poetry. Keeping a diary seeks to keep a date for the fulfillment of literary aspirations. The chapter titles hover over the schizoid protagonist's disorientation, spelling out the uncanny continuity between the days or dates of his stay and the dates of historical battles that in the game are not yet lost or won.

Something like paranoia prompts him to breach the privacy of the apartment in which the ailing hotel owner is holed up. Berger walks in on a Grand Inquisitor scene. While the hotel owner judges that Berger's current adversary in the game is the devil, the player opts out of the Faustian allegory (although he names Goethe his favorite poet) and recognizes in the gray eminence's profile Don Quixote instead. The scene propped up by literary references rededicates the game-changing as play of the imagination no longer constrained by the compulsive not-seeing of traumatic history. He turns his back on the game and what remains is the diary, which by the end is coextensive with the novel.

Notes

1 This is a possible interpretation of *The Postmodern Condition* (1974).

2 Kathy Acker, *Don Quixote Which Was a Dream* (New York: Grove Press, 1986). Page references are given in the text.

3 *2666*, trans. Natasha Wimmer (New York: Farrar, Straus and Giroux, 2008). Page references are given in the text.

4 *By Night in Chile*, trans. Chris Andrews (New York: New Directions Books, 2003). Page numbers are given in the text.

5 Bolaño revisited and expanded on the closing case in *Nazi Literature in the Americas* in a subsequent novella, *Distant Star*, trans. Chris Andrews (New York: New Directions Books, 2004). The poet's name is Ramirez Hoffman in the compendium of Nazi literature. Page references are to the longer revision and are given in the text.

6 *The Third Reich*, trans. Natasha Wimmer (New York: Farrar, Straus and Giroux, 2011). Page references are given in the text. The book packs the proviso that all the characters, organizations and events portrayed in the novel are either products of the author's imagination or are used fictitiously.

7 Sans the board game this is the gist of my Bond reading in *SPECTRE* (Fort Wayne: Anti-Oedipus Press, 2013).

Index

Note: page numbers followed by n refer to notes.

For Product Safety Concerns and Information please contact our EU representative GPSR@taylorandfrancis.com Taylor & Francis Verlag GmbH, Kaufingerstraße 24, 80331 München, Germany